THE NURSE'S GUIDE TO FLUID AND ELECTROLYTE BALANCE

The Nurse's Guide Series

The Nurse's Guide to Fluid and Electrolyte Balance
The Nurse's Guide to Diagnostic Procedures
The Nurse's Guide to Cardiac Surgery and Nursing Care

THE NURSE'S GUIDE TO FLUID AND ELECTROLYTE BALANCE

AUDREY BURGESS, R.N., B.S., M.A.
*New York University
Assistant Director of Nursing,
Harlem Hospital Center School of Nursing*

McGRAW-HILL BOOK COMPANY
A Blakiston Publication
NEW YORK ST. LOUIS SAN FRANCISCO DÜSSELDORF
LONDON MEXICO PANAMA RIO DE JANEIRO
SINGAPORE SYDNEY TORONTO

This book is dedicated to Dr. Barbara Howell for her inestimable assistance in its development; to the students in the School of Nursing at The State University of New York at Buffalo who struggled through the lectures and clinical experiences which were later developed into the content found herein; and to the girls in the secretarial pool who struggled with my handwriting during the preparation of those lectures and later notes.

This book was set in Optima by Monotype Composition Company, Inc., and printed on permanent paper and bound by Vail-Ballou Press, Inc. The designer was J. E. O'Connor; the drawings were done by Peter Ng. The editors were Joseph J. Brehm, Bernice Heller, and Sally Mobley. Annette Wentz supervised production.

THE NURSE'S GUIDE TO FLUID
AND ELECTROLYTE BALANCE

Copyright © 1970 by McGraw-Hill, Inc. All rights reserved. Printed in the United States of America. No part of this publication may be reproduced, stored in a retrieval system, or transmitted, in any form or by any means, electronic, mechanical, photocopying, recording, or otherwise, without the prior written permission of the publisher.

Library of Congress Catalog Card Number 71-133390
07-008954-X

6789l0ll2 MUMU 987654

PREFACE

I suppose that to some persons reading a book, it is interesting to know why the author wrote the book. At any rate, once having written it, one is urged by one's publishers to tell in the preface the reasons "why."

One writes because one has to. An individual becomes interested in a subject. He studies it. If, in his search for the truth concerning the subject of his interest, he discovers that other persons have not said enough to tell him what he wants to know, he begins to formulate his own truth. At this point, he begins to feel that he has a statement to make, in a particular way, that has not been made before. He begins to make that statement in speeches, conversations, lectures, memoranda—whatever the medium afforded by his daily occupation. The end result is a written statement and an attempt to get the statement published in order to share with others what he has to say. The form of the writing may be prose or poetry; the subject may be electrolytes or love. But neither form nor subject is the important element in writing; rather, what is important is what the author has to say.

This book addresses itself to the subject of fluid and electrolytes. I wrote it because I thought I had something to say that had not adequately, fully, or clearly been said in this particular way before. This reason holds most vigorously in those parts of the book dealing with the nurse's role in maintenance of fluid and electrolyte balance and in regard to the clinical teaching of the subject.

Over a period of seven years of teaching in two-, three-, and four-year nursing programs, it was my experience that the literature describing the physiology of fluid and electrolyte balance was often either too complex or oversimplified for the nursing student. Further, there were few concrete relationships established in the literature between the *physiology* and what the nurse *saw, did,* and *said* in the process of patient care. For fifteen years it has been my conviction that the teaching of nursing from a disease entity orientation resulted in boring redundancy and frequently missed the most important part of the message to the student, i.e., *what* is the precise nurse-patient interaction appropriate to a particular situation and *how* is that interaction similar to or different from other nursing approaches used in other situations.

Thus it has been my intent in making my statement to demonstrate that the maintenance of fluid and electrolyte balance is a nursing objective common to the care of patients in a variety of clinical states; that nursing approaches designed to meet that common objective are basically similar without regard to the cause of the specific problem. I have attempted to unify understanding of physiological and pathophysiological responses of the body in the maintenance of fluid and electrolyte balance with identified nursing observations, assessments, and approaches.

It is my hope that the broad base of similarities in the aforementioned areas will serve as a background of common elements against which specific differences become more evident under special circumstances.

Audrey Burgess

CONTENTS

PREFACE v

PART ONE
THE PHYSIOLOGY OF BODY FLUID AND ELECTROLYTES

Chapter

1 Introduction 3
2 Characteristics and Functions of Body Fluid and Electrolytes 7
3 Regulation of Body Fluid and Electrolytes and Acid-base Balance 24
4 Avenues of Gains and Losses of Body Fluid and Electrolytes 34
5 Body Responses to Changes in Body Fluid, Electrolytes, and Acid-base Balance 42

PART TWO
NURSING INTERVENTION IN MAINTENANCE AND RESTORATION OF FLUID AND ELECTROLYTE BALANCE

Chapter

6 The Nurse's Role in Observation and Assessment 55
7 The Nurse's Role in Helping to Meet Patient and Family Needs 71
8 The Nurse's Role in Relation to That of Other Health Team Members 82

PART THREE
APPROACH TO CLINICAL STUDY FOR THE STUDENT AND THE TEACHER

Chapter

9 A Problem-solving Approach to Nursing Assessment 93
10 Suggestions for Clinical Teaching 99

INDEX 115

PART ONE
THE PHYSIOLOGY OF BODY FLUID AND ELECTROLYTES

ONE
INTRODUCTION

A review of the clinical states frequently associated with fluid and electrolyte imbalance reveals 65 percent of them to be conditions which the nurse commonly encounters in patients for whom she provides daily care (see Table 1-1). Most of the states listed on Bland's table cause sodium and water imbalance. One study has shown 20 percent of the adult patients in one large hospital to have had low serum potassium levels. Inadequate intake was found to be the most common cause of these particular low potassium levels.[1] Recovery rooms, intensive care units, and coronary care units, which have markedly increased in number in recent years, provide care for a variety of patients in whom the balance of fluid and electrolyte is a central medical and nursing problem. The trend toward early discharge sends patients home on regimens

[1] B. Surawica et al., "Clinical Manifestations of Hypopotassemia," *American Journal of Medical Science,* 233:603, 1957.

Table 1–1 *Clinical States Frequently Producing Electrolyte or Fluid Imbalance*

I. Sodium and water depletion, with only water replacement or inadequate sodium replacement
   A. Gastrointestinal secretion losses
      1. Vomiting
      2. Diarrhea
      3. Gastric or intestinal intubation, drainage, and/or suction
      4. Exchange resins—may inhibit absorption of dietary Na^+ and augment a depletion and low $(Na^+)_e$ from other causes; not in itself a potent cause
   B. Skin losses
      1. Excessive sweating
      2. Burn areas with loss of extracellular water (ECW) through damaged skin; often underestimated in magnitude
      3. Skin wounds with exudate containing much water and electrolyte
      4. Exudative dermatologic lesions
   C. Renal losses of Na^+ and water
      1. Drug effects
         a. Mercurial diuresis
         b. Acetazolamide (Diamox)
         c. Excess anion load, e.g., ammonium chloride (NH_4Cl)
      2. Intrinsic renal disease
         a. Na^+-losing nephritis (uncommon)
         b. Diuretic phase of acute renal insufficiency
         c. Nephrosis
         d. Chronic renal insufficiency with renal acidosis
      3. Metabolic losses, osmotic diuresis
         a. Starvation ketosis
         b. Diabetic acidosis with glucose as the loading solute increasing rate of urine flow and with it the rate of Na^+ excretion
         c. Urea as the leading solute when used as a diuretic
         d. Metabolic acidosis of any etiology—H^+- and NH_3-forming mechanism saturated and Na^+ excreted over and above this
      4. Endocrinologic disease
         a. Adrenocortical insufficiency
            i. Primary
            ii. Secondary to panhypopituitarism

Table 1-1 *Clinical States Frequently Producing Electrolyte or Fluid Imbalance (continued)*

		b.	Hypercortisonism on withdrawal of adrenocorticosteroid therapy
		5.	Cerebral salt wastage, producing symptoms in contradistinction to asymptomatic hyponatremia
	D.	Losses from serous cavities	
		1.	Paracentesis in ascites with free access to water afterward
		2.	Thoracentesis—usually occurs with repeated withdrawals
		3.	Surgical drainage of any large cavity
	E.	Translocation of extracellular water	
		1.	Severe urticaria
		2.	Extensive sunburn
		3.	Rapid re-formation of ascites
		4.	Milk leg, massive
II.	Excessive water intake with intact or increased total body Na$^+$		
	A.	Abnormality in water and Na$^+$ excretion associated with:	
		1.	Portal cirrhosis
		2.	Congestive failure of the circulation
		3.	Chronic or acute renal insufficiency
	B.	Water intoxication	
		1.	Water administration greater than maximal renal excretory rate for water
		2.	Water administration when ADH is very active
		3.	Excess water administered during anuria
III.	Asymptomatic hyponatremia—intracellular loss of osmolarity		
	A.	Advanced pulmonary disease	
	B.	Cachexia and malnutrition	
	C.	Advanced physiological aging	
	D.	Portal cirrhosis	
IV.	Na$^+$ movement into intracellular water (ICW) with water movement in extracellular water in metabolic alkalosis (H$^+$ and NA$^+$ replacing one K$^+$ in cell)		
V.	Extracellular water hyperosmolarity		
	A.	Infusion of solution which remains in extracellular water and does not readily diffuse into the cells; e.g., glucose, mannitol (not urea) may augment urinary losses of Na$^+$	

Source: John Bland, *Clinical Metabolism of Body Water and Electrolytes,* W. B. Saunders Company, Philadelphia; 1963.

of diuretics and adrenocorticosteroid medications or with other provisions for self-care which may affect fluid and electrolyte balance. The whole point, obviously, is that in order to assist patients, we as nurses need to understand what is meant by fluid and electrolyte balance and imbalance. In addition, we must clearly recognize and carry out those independent and dependent nurse actions which aid the patient in maintenance of fluid and electrolyte balance.

This monograph reviews some basic physiological and clinical facts regarding fluid and electrolyte balance and then goes on to a brief discussion of the types of conditions which cause imbalances. Common objective and subjective symptoms are identified and classified to aid memorization and to facilitate understanding. The nurse's role in the observation and assessment of patient needs, in dealing with patient and family needs, and in relation to other health team members is discussed. Her role with respect to fluid replacement therapy as well as the administration of diuretic drug therapy is considered. Diagnostic tests are reviewed in relation to normal ranges. Patient situations with study questions and a section on suggestions for clinical teaching are also features of this monograph.

TWO
CHARACTERISTICS AND FUNCTIONS OF BODY FLUID AND ELECTROLYTES

GENERAL CHARACTERISTICS OF BODY FLUID

The body is composed primarily of water in which are dissolved the substances essential to life. Water accounts for 57 to 60 percent of an adult's body weight and 75 to 80 percent of an infant's weight (see Figure 2–1). This is one reason why daily weighing of the patient is mandatory when the physician suspects the patient to be retaining or losing fluid. Such instances come readily to mind, for example, the patient with congestive heart failure, burns, ulcerative colitis, or uremia.

The amount of body water is influenced by the relative proportions of different tissues present in the individual's body. Fat contains little water; therefore, the more obese the individual, the smaller his body water content in comparison to his size. This is one reason obese patients are considered poor surgical risks.

Normally the amount of body fluid decreases with age (see

BODY COMPOSITION
■ WATER
▦ FATS + FAT FREE SOLIDS

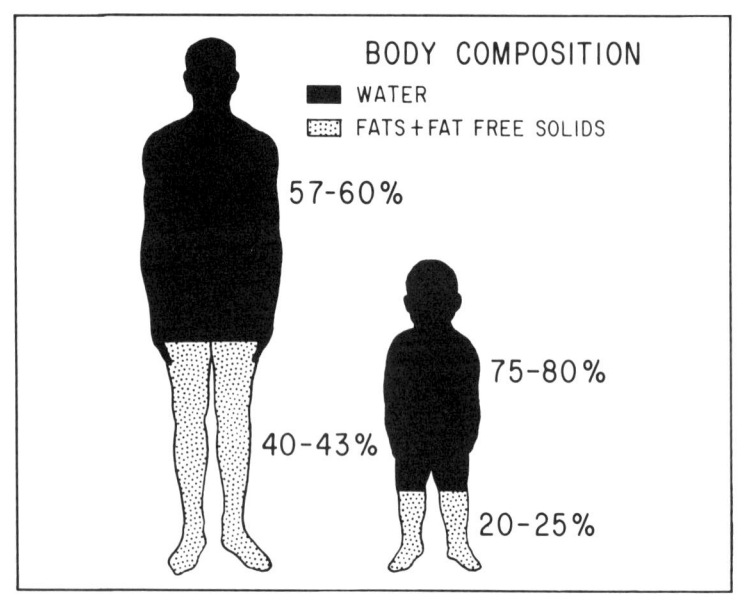

57-60%

75-80%

40-43%

20-25%

Figure 2–1 *Body composition.*

Figure 2–2). Thus older patients have less fluid reserves to draw upon when their fluid intake is decreased or a loss of fluid occurs. The aged patient's decrease in extracellular fluid reserve is one reason he may be unable to withstand the rigors of surgery. Infants' weights reflect a high water content. Their high metabolic rate causes a rapid turnover of water which is almost three times the exchange of adults. Witness the frequency with which they urinate and defecate or notice their tiny, shiny, perspiring faces when they are eating. This rapid turnover of water in infants together with the relatively large amount of water found in their extracellular space and the inability of their kidneys to concentrate urine causes infants to have varying water needs from adults. These factors also result in infants being more susceptible to the untoward effects of increases or decreases of body fluids.

BODY WATER CONTENT

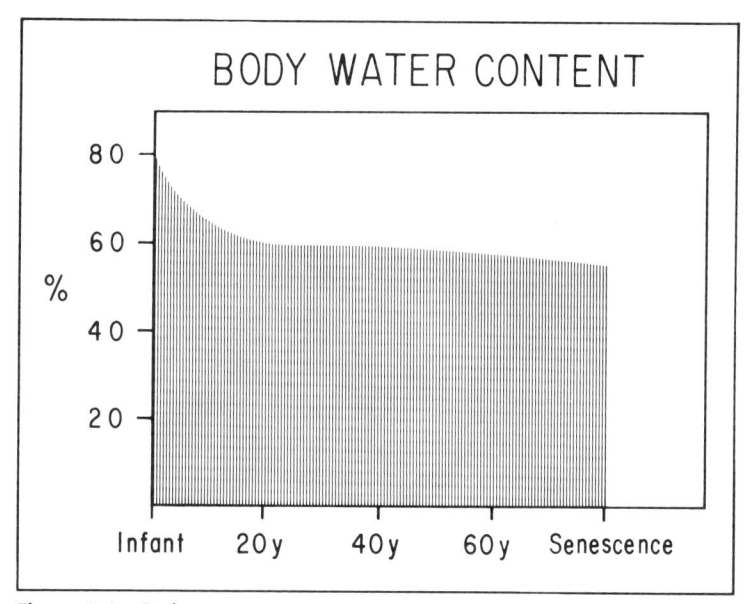

Figure 2–2 *Body water content.*

The fluid of the body provides the essential environment in which the chemical and physical reactions requisite to life can take place. For example, a fluid medium is necessary for the transportation of nutrients to and waste products from the cells.

The largest amount of body fluid in adults is found inside the cells and is known as *intracellular* fluid. In contrast to fluid found outside the cells it is relatively stable, that is, it does not move into and out of the cell readily. The *extracellular* fluid, although less quantitatively than intracellular fluid, moves freely between the microcirculatory beds, capillaries, small venules, and interstitial spaces between the cells.

Blood plasma, interstitial fluid, and intraocular and cerebrospinal fluid are all part of the extracellular fluid.

MOVEMENT OF BODY FLUID

Diffusion

Body fluids and their dissolved constituents move between the microcirculatory beds, interstitial spaces, and cells by means of different variations of the basic process of diffusion. Diffusion, you recall, is the movement of molecules or ions from areas of greater concentration of the particular substance to areas of lesser concentration of that molecule or ion. Diffusion from areas of greater concentration to areas of lesser concentration is called *diffusion along the concentration gradient*. Diffusion along the concentration gradient through living tissue occurs in three ways. Sometimes the molecules are small enough to pass through spaces between cells or to squeeze through small holes in the cell membrane.

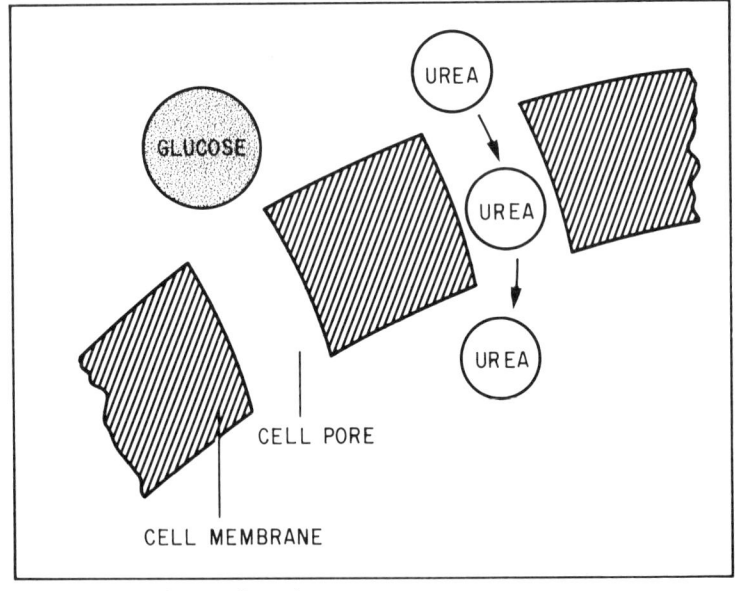

Figure 2-3 *Diffusion through pores.*

These holes are called *pores* (see Figure 2–3). Urea is an example of such a molecule.

Some substances such as alcohol and oxygen are capable of dissolving into the fatty part of the cell membrane, moving through, into, and across the cell, then out the other side (see Figure 2–4).

Other substances are diffused through the cell membrane into the cell by becoming chemically combined with a carrier substance on the surface of the cell membrane. The new chemical combination thus formed is capable of dissolving into the fatty part of the membrane and diffusing inside the cell. Once inside the cell, the new chemical combination undergoes a reversal of the original chemical change. The carrier substances return to the cell membrane while the carried substance is released inside the

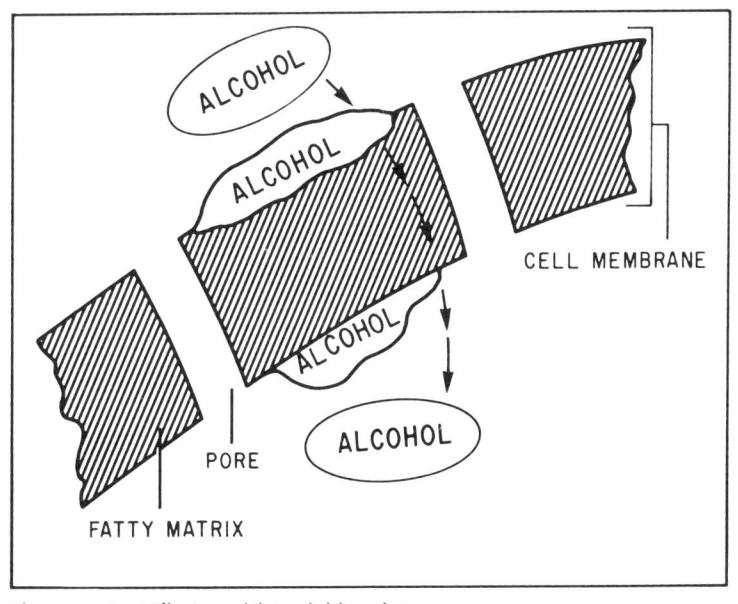

Figure 2–4 *Diffusion of fat-soluble substances.*

cell. This process is known as *facilitated diffusion* (see Figure 2-5). Glucose passes into cells in this manner.

Diffusion of all three types described occurs in the direction of the concentration gradient until an equilibrium is reached between the amounts of a particular kind of solute on either side of the semipermeable membrane. This membrane can be the cell membrane or the capillary wall. The capillary wall is not a single membrane. However, the thin flat endothelial cells and the spaces between them act as a semipermeable membrane between the vascular system and the interstitial spaces.

Sometimes it is necessary for substances such as sodium to be moved through a cell membrane against the concentration gradient (that is, *toward* an area of greater concentration of the particular substance) (see Figure 2-6). This happens in the renal tubules of the kidney. The process by which a substance moves

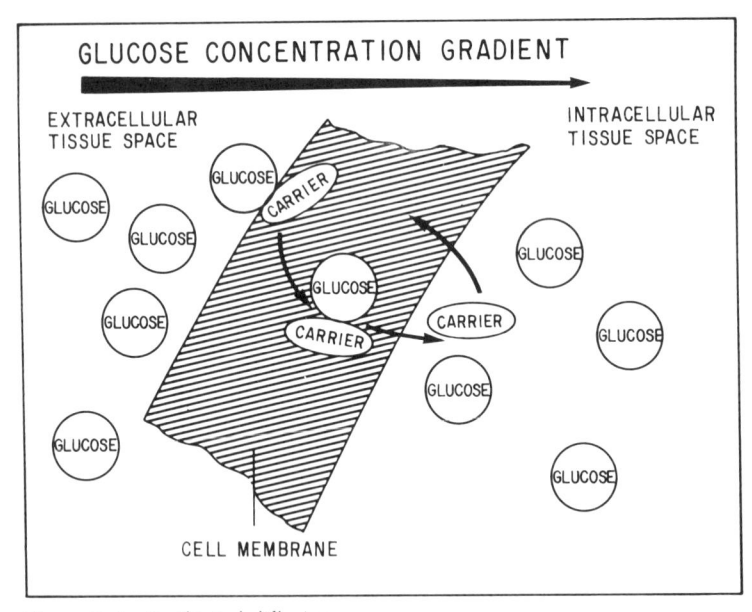

Figure 2-5 *Facilitated diffusion.*

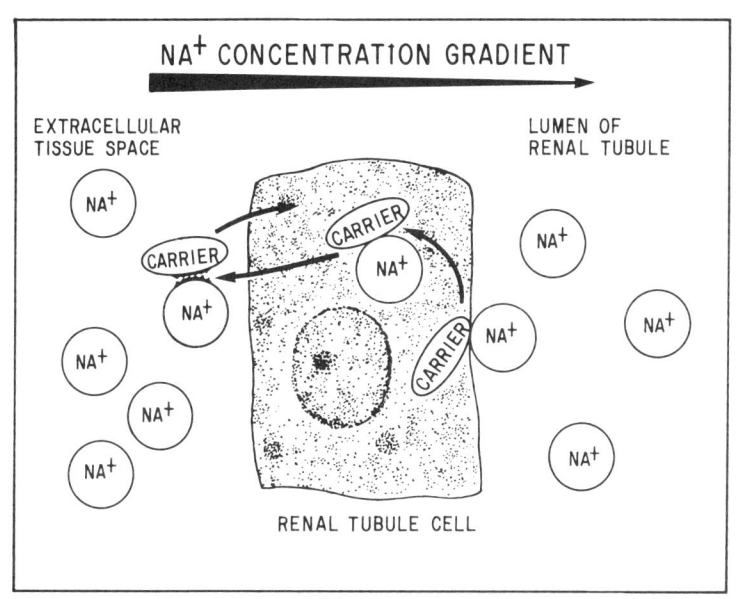

Figure 2–6 *Active transport.*

into or across a cell against the concentration gradient is known as *active transport* and is similar to facilitated diffusion in all respects except that it occurs *against* the concentration gradient.

Osmosis

Water molecules when separated by a semipermeable membrane are constantly moving back and forth across the membrane. The movement of water across a semipermeable membrane is called *osmosis* (see Figure 2–7). During the process of osmosis water is diffusing toward the area of lesser concentration of *water molecules*. However, since the concentration of a solution is expressed in terms of the amount of solute dissolved in the solvent, the solution on the right side of Figure 2–7 is considered the "concentrated" solution. Under laboratory conditions osmosis con-

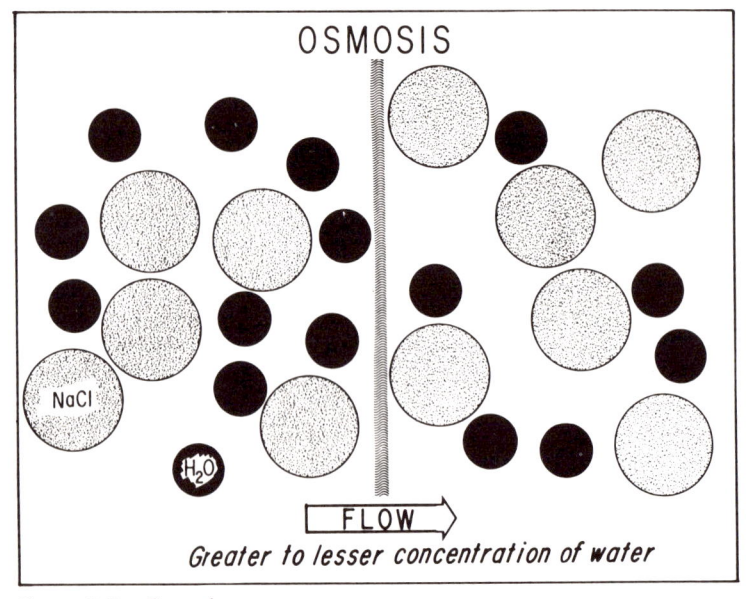

Figure 2-7 *Osmosis.*

tinues until the pressure resisting the inflow of water molecules (hydrostatic pressure) is great enough to bring diffusion to a standstill. This resisting pressure, which accumulates when osmosis is demonstrated under laboratory conditions, is the pressure due to the weight of a column of the water and for this reason is called *hydrostatic pressure*. In the human organism this resistance to osmosis exerted by the body fluid is also called hydrostatic pressure, but there are other factors which also affect the direction and rate of osmosis. Among these factors are body temperature and hydrostatic pressure both within the capillary lumen and in the surrounding interstitial spaces. The kinds and amounts of solutes present in body fluid also have effects on the movement of body water. By chemically interacting with water, the solutes in a water solution determine the concentration of those water molecules which are free to move by osmosis. The direction of osmosis

CHARACTERISTICS AND FUNCTIONS OF BODY FLUID AND ELECTROLYTES   15

of water is toward the area with the least free water molecules and the greatest concentration of solutes. The degree to which the solutes can affect the movement of the water is called their osmotic power. Nonprotein solutes exert *crystalloid* osmotic power, whereas proteins exert *colloid* osmotic power. Body fluid and replacement solutions are described in terms of their osmotic power or osmolarity (that is, the ability of their solutes to draw water or give up water across a semipermeable membrane). A more familiar term denoting their osmotic power is tonicity. When referring to the tonicity of a replacement fluid one is talking about the degree to which the replacement fluid will allow movement of water in and out of body cells.

Isotonic replacement solutions, such as normal saline (see Figure 2–8), have concentrations of water and salt equal to those usually found in the body. In isotonic solutions the concentration

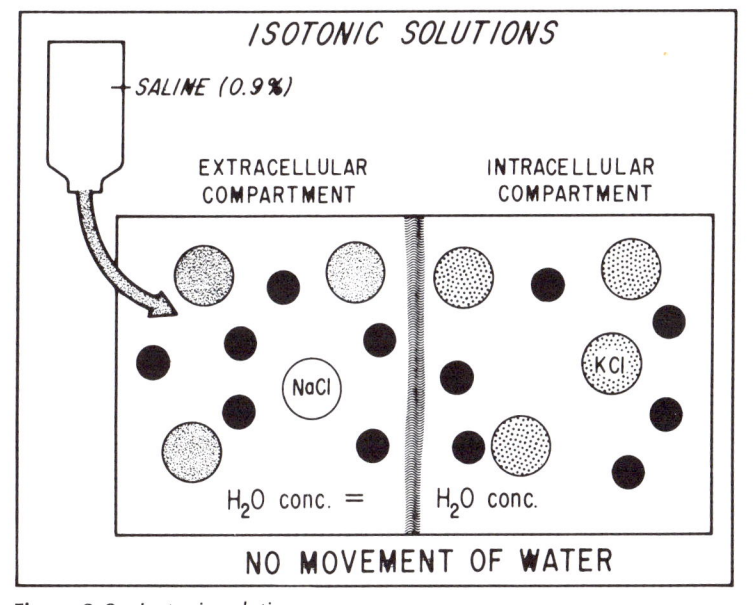

Figure 2–8 *Isotonic solutions.*

of water molecules free to move by osmosis is equal to free water molecules found in isotonic body fluid. Thus, replacement solutions which are isotonic have drawing power for water equal to normal body fluids and will not pass into or draw water from the cells. Isotonic replacement solutions are administered to patients who have lost fluid from the cardiovascular system, as in hemorrhage, or who have experienced rapid loss of fluid from some other part of the extracellular fluid compartment, as in vomiting or sweating. The isotonic solution circulates and diffuses in the extracellular fluid compartment, thus restoring the balance of fluid between the outside and inside of the cells. If isotonic solutions are not given to the patient who needs them or if the patient's losses outstrip the rate at which they can be replaced, fluid will shift from the inside of the cells into the extracellular fluid compartment. Intracellular dehydration can then be said to be present.

Hypotonic replacement solutions are solutions which have concentrations of free water molecules greater than the concentration of free water molecules inside the cells. If hypotonic solutions are injected into a dehydrated person who is experiencing loss of intracellular fluid, the hypotonic solution will give up the water molecules the cells need to return to isotonic equilibrium (see Figure 2–9).

When intracellular dehydration occurs, the water content of the body fluid inside the cell may be so depleted that solutions which are isotonic and even hypertonic to *normal* body fluid are, relatively speaking, potentially hypotonic and give up their water to the dehydrated cells. This is seen when 2.5 percent glucose in 0.45 or 0.5 percent saline is given to adults to replace intracellular fluid loss. Again, 5 percent or 2.5 percent glucose in 0.33 percent or 0.25 percent saline is given to infants requiring similar hydration. Hypotonic or potentially hypotonic solutions must be given at slower rates than isotonic solutions because a sudden shift of fluid into the cells may cause shock and cerebral edema. The shock occurs from the sudden loss of blood volume. The sudden influx of water into cells causes edema of the cells, including those

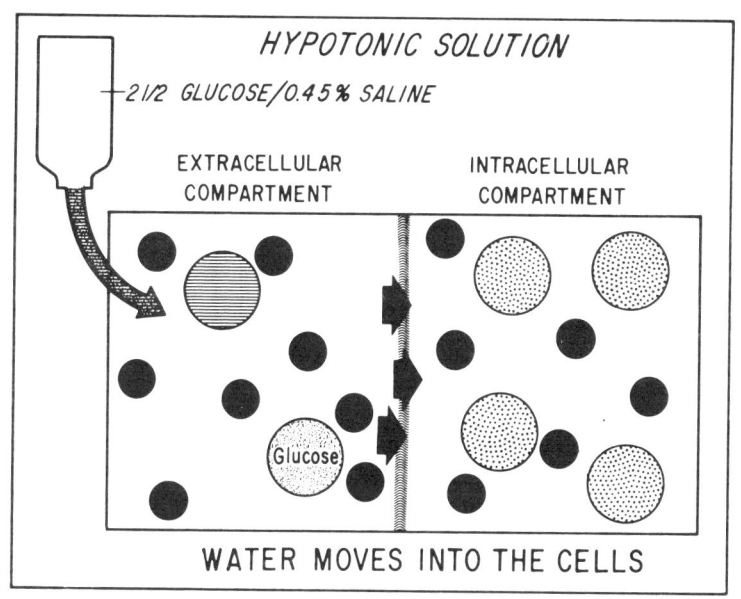

CHARACTERISTICS AND FUNCTIONS OF BODY FLUID AND ELECTROLYTES

Figure 2-9 *Relatively hypotonic solution to dehydrated intracellular fluid.*

of the brain. Shock and cerebral edema may combine to cause death of the patient.

Often cerebral edema occurs in patients as a corollary of some other clinical state such as traumatic head injury. In this condition and others in which cells retain water, hypertonic solutions may be administered to the patient. Hypertonic solutions having a lower concentration of free water molecules than that of the body fluid inside the cells will draw water from the cells (see Figure 2-10). Some common hypertonic replacement solutions are 50 percent glucose in water, 10 percent fructose in water, 10 percent dextrose in water, and 5 percent dextrose in lactated Ringer's solution. Hypertonic solutions must also be given more slowly than isotonic solutions. As with hypotonic solutions, rapid administration of hypertonic solutions may cause a sudden shift of fluid.

HYPERTONIC SOLUTION
50% GLUCOSE IN WATER

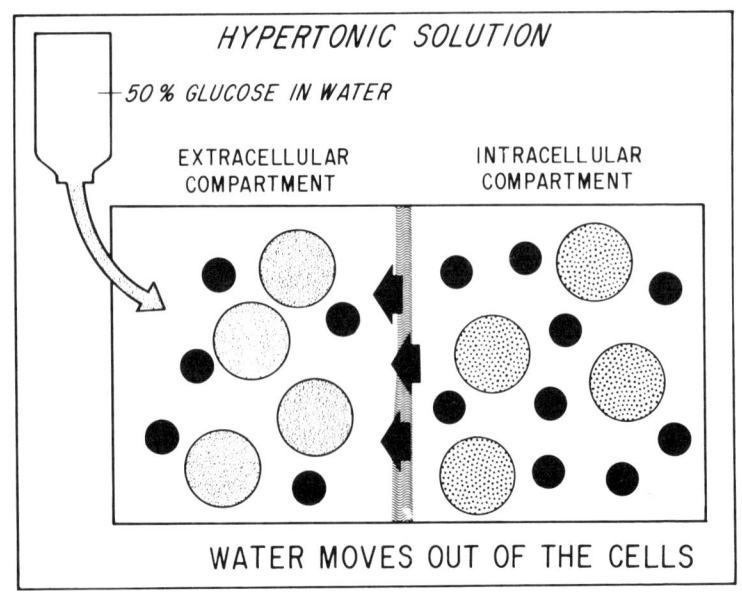

EXTRACELLULAR COMPARTMENT — INTRACELLULAR COMPARTMENT

WATER MOVES OUT OF THE CELLS

Figure 2–10 *Hypertonic solutions.*

However, this shift is from within the cells to interstitial space and ultimately to the vascular system. The overload of fluid in the circulation created by this sudden shift of fluid from the cells can cause cardiac failure, pulmonary edema, and death.

Hydrostatic and Colloid Osmotic Pressure

Hydrostatic pressure as defined by Guyton is the pressure of a fluid resulting from the weight of the water molecules in the fluid.[1] Oncotic pressure, or colloid osmotic pressure, refers to the osmotic pull of proteins in the body fluids. The pushing power of intracapillary blood pressure (hydrostatic pressure) and the pulling

[1] Arthur Guyton, *A Textbook of Medical Physiology*, 2d ed., W. B. Saunders Company, Philadelphia, 1961, p. 370.

power of proteins (colloid osmotic pressure) in the capillaries and the capillary interstitial spaces aid in the movement of body fluid into and out of these small vessels. There are factors other than the weight of the water molecules which also affect the degree of hydrostatic pressure in a closed system of tubes such as the cardiovascular system or infusion fluid and tubing connected to the cardiovascular system. One such factor is the height of the column of liquid in which the pressure is being measured. For example, in the standing human, hydrostatic pressure of blood in the arteries and veins of the lower extremities is greater than that in the vessels of the upper extremities. Muscular movement and the vein valves help overcome the effects of the high hydrostatic pressure in the extremities. However, when stasis of blood occurs in the lower extremities, the push of vascular hydrostatic pressure becomes so great that fluid is forced out of the capillaries into the tissues, and edema occurs. Prolonged bed rest, immobilization, and congestive heart failure are all instances in which stasis of blood in the lower extremities can lead to increased hydrostatic pressure and subsequent edema.

The size of the cross-section of the lumen of a vessel with respect to the volume of blood within the vessel also affects the hydrostatic pressure. A decreased luminal cross section with no change in blood volume will increase the hydrostatic pressure. The anatomical structure of microcirculatory vessels leading to and from the capillaries (that is, narrow at the arterial end, wider at the venule end) favors a high hydrostatic pressure at the arterial end of the microcirculatory vessels and thus the movement of body fluid out of them to the interstitial spaces. As the amount of intracapillary fluid diminishes in volume and the luminal cross section increases in size, the hydrostatic pressure decreases. Thus, toward the venous end of the microcirculatory vessels, the interstitial fluid is drawn back into the blood vessel by the osmotic pull of the blood proteins, which remain constant in amount and osmolarity throughout the capillary.

In the glomerular capillary the constant outward movement of fluid and solutes is favored by the unique structural arrangement of the capillary anastomosing on either end with an arteriole. Other factors affect the exchange of fluid across the capillary membrane, but the interaction of the pull of colloid osmotic pressure and the push of hydrostatic pressure inside and around the microcirculatory vessels is the major force.[2, 3]

Osmosis and hydrostatic pressure are important to understand because the combined interaction of osmotic pull and hydrostatic push determines the direction of body water movement into and out of the capillaries.

Diffusion, osmosis, and hydrostatic pressure have been discussed because these three biophysical mechanisms are functional throughout the human body. Body fluid, in its liquid state, and body cells and interstitial tissue, in their semiliquid state, provide the milieu for the constant transport of gases and nutrients from the outside of the body to cells and the transferral of waste products from the cells to the exterior of the body. Fluid and electrolyte balance in the human organism depends upon the exchange of solutes and fluids between the intracellular and extracellular compartments of the body; this exchange is dependent upon the biophysical mechanisms discussed. Anything which interferes with these biophysical mechanisms will lead to a derangement of the supply of gases, nutrients, and water to the cells and removal of wastes from the cells. This deranged physiological state is described as *fluid and electrolyte imbalance.*

CHARACTERISTICS, FUNCTIONS, AND MEASUREMENT OF ELECTROLYTES

Substances which have the property of breaking down in water into positively or negatively charged particles are called *electrolytes* or *ions*. The positively charged electrolytes are called cations (see Figure 2–11), whereas negatively charged electrolytes are called anions. Some substances, such as organic acids, proteins,

[2] Guyton, op. cit., pp. 52–63.
[3] Robert Berne and Matthew N. Levy, *Cardiovascular Physiology,* The C. V. Mosby Company, St. Louis, 1967, pp. 104–107.

Figure 2–11

Cations		Anions	
	Electrolytes		
Potassium	K⁺	Chloride	Cl⁻
Sodium	Na⁺	Sulphate	SO₄⁻⁻
Magnesium	Mg⁺⁺	Phosphate	HPO₄⁻⁻
Calcium	Ca⁺⁺	Bicarbonate	HCO₃⁻
	Other Electrochemical Substances		
Carbonic acid	H₂CO₃	Proteins	
		Organic acids	

and carbonic acid, are not, strictly speaking, electrolytes but have the potential of dissociating into electrically charged particles or of having an electrical pull. These substances are also called electrolytes.

All types of electrolytes are found both inside and outside the cells. However, extracellular fluid has large amounts of sodium chloride and bicarbonate electrolytes. Intracellular fluid contains large amounts of potassium, phosphates, sulfates, and protein electrolytes. Although the electrochemical composition of the fluid inside and outside the cell varies in the amount of different electrolytes, the total positive and negative charges on the inside and outside of the cell are normally equal.

Electrolytes are measured in terms of their ability to go into electrochemical combination with other electrolytes (see Figure 2–12). Opposite electrical charges attract one another. The doctor needs to know how many electrolytes of a particular substance are available in each 1000 cc of body fluid to attract oppositely charged electrolytes of another substance. The laboratory report tells him this when the electrolytes are reported in milliequivalents per liter (see Figure 2–13).

Electrolytes function in maintaining water distribution in the body, a balanced degree of neuromuscular irritability, and the

MILLIEQUIVALENT IS:

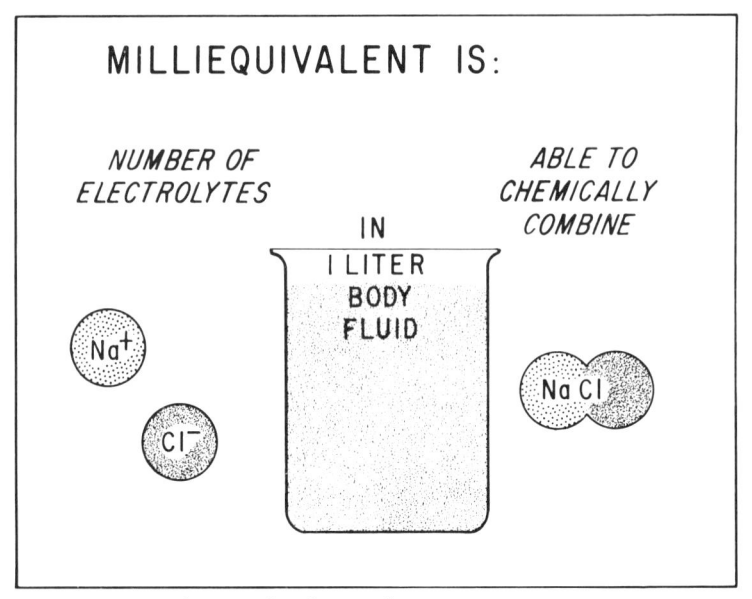

NUMBER OF ELECTROLYTES IN 1 LITER BODY FLUID *ABLE TO CHEMICALLY COMBINE*

Na+   Cl−   Na Cl

Figure 2–12 *Definition of milliequivalent.*

acid-base balance of the body. The role of electrolytes in movement of fluid about the body was described in relation to crystalloid osmotic pressure in the previous chapter. The role of electrolytes in acid-base balance will be discussed in the next chapter.

Some cells of the body are capable of transmitting electrochemical impulses along their membranes. These cells include nerve, muscle, and probably glandular cells. As a result of the spread of the electrochemical impulse nerve cells transmit impulses, from one to another, sending messages to various portions of the brain, or back to muscle. The electrochemical impulse from the nerve cell stimulates the muscle cell to move by causing a change in its electrochemical state. Glandular cells are thought to respond to electrochemical changes in their cell membrane by secreting whatever substance is peculiar to the gland.

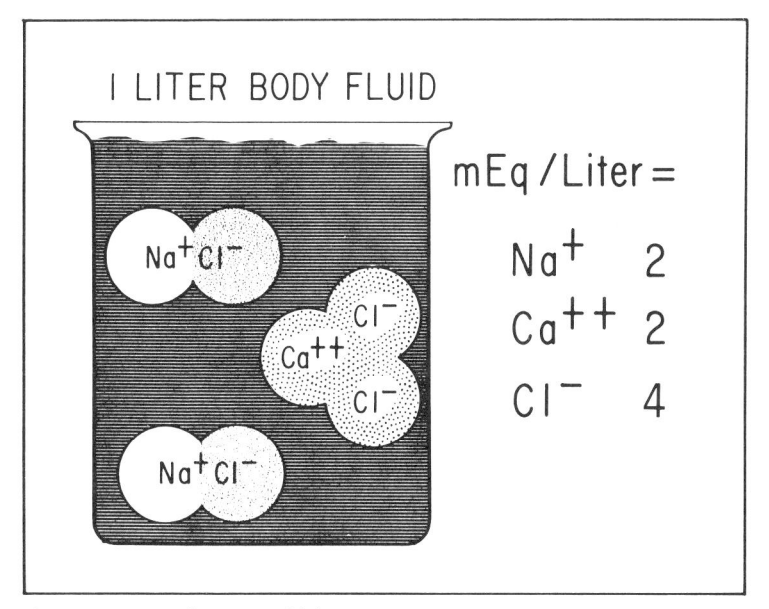

Figure 2-13 *Explanation of laboratory report.*

All cells have higher potassium concentrations intracellularly under normal resting conditions; sodium is usually found in greater quantities outside the cell. Differing stimuli may cause sodium ions to begin to diffuse into the cell and potassium ions to diffuse out of the cell. This movement of positively charged ions back and forth causes a change in the cell membrane which becomes the electrochemical impulse described in the foregoing paragraph. The stimuli precipitating the change may be chemical in nature, such as the release of acetylcholine by a nerve fiber at its junction with a muscle. Mechanical stimulation, such as the prick of a pin, can provide the stimulus to a nerve fiber. Other electrolytes also have a role in the maintenance of balance in neuromuscular irritability.[4]

[4] Guyton, op. cit., pp. 217–227.

THREE
REGULATION OF BODY FLUID AND ELECTROLYTES AND ACID-BASE BALANCE

RENAL REGULATION

Although the lungs are operant in regulation of the amount of carbon dioxide in the circulating blood, the concentration of nonprotein constituents of body fluid is controlled primarily by the kidneys. Body fluid volume is also controlled by the kidneys. Each kidney is comprised of approximately one million functional units called nephrons. Each nephron functions independently of the other nephrons, but all normal nephrons function in the same manner. Thus, to discuss the function of one normal nephron in the regulation of volume and concentration of body fluids is to describe the function of the normal kidney in these respects. The kidney plays a central role in the maintenance of fluid and electrolyte balance. It is important that the nurse understand that role in order to provide intelligent nursing intervention.

The nephron is made up of a system of renal tubules in close proximity to arterioles, capillaries, and venules (see Figure 3–1).

BODY FLUID, ELECTROLYTES, AND ACID-BASE BALANCE

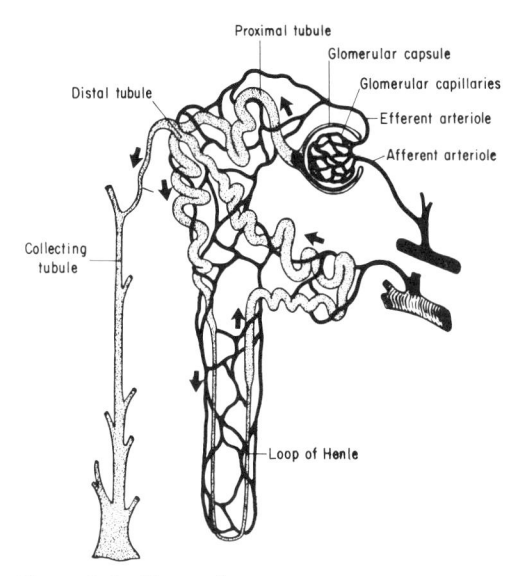

Figure 3–1 *The nephron.*

One end of the nephron known as the *glomerular capsule* encloses a coil of capillaries called the *glomerular tuft* or *capillaries*. The other end of the nephron empties into the collecting tubules of the kidneys.

The structure of the glomerular capillaries favors constant filtration of body fluid and dissolved substances from the blood into the renal tubules. This composite liquid, known as the *glomerular filtrate,* is identical in composition to blood plasma with one exception: blood plasma contains proteins which are too large to filter into the tubules. As the filtrate passes through the renal tubules, the dissolved substances and varying amounts of the fluid are reabsorbed first into the interstitial spaces surrounding the tubules and then from the interstitial spaces into the blood vessels surrounding the renal tubules. Electrolytes such as sodium and potassium are reabsorbed by active transport through the tubular cells which act in response to hormonal substances in the blood.

Other solutes are reabsorbed depending on the body's needs and the blood levels of these substances. Water is reabsorbed by osmosis in response to the degree of tonicity of the interstitial body fluid surrounding the kidney tubules and in response to a humoral substance called *antidiuretic hormone* (ADH). The remaining filtrate is then excreted as urine.

It is believed that the supraoptic nuclei cells in the hypothalamus both secrete ADH and regulate, by neural impulses, its release from its storage place in the posterior pituitary gland. Another theory hypothesizes that the supraoptic cells merely transmit impulses and that in response the cells in the posterior pituitary gland both secrete and release ADH.[1,2] Whichever theory is

[1] Arthur Guyton, *A Textbook of Medical Physiology*, 3d ed., W. B. Saunders Company, Philadelphia, 1966, pp. 1045–1047.
[2] Harry Statland, *Fluid and Electrolytes in Practice*, 2d ed., J. B. Lippincott Company, Philadelphia, 1957, pp. 20–22.

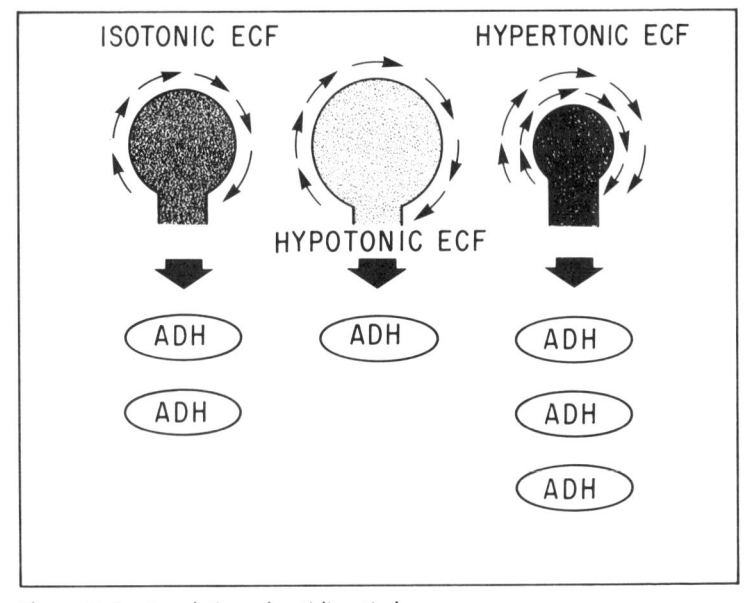

Figure 3–2 *Regulation of antidiuretic hormone.*

correct, it is known that osmoreceptor cells in the hypothalamus allow for a constant secretion of ADH which increases or decreases in relation to the tonicity of surrounding body fluids. ADH is secreted at a rate related to neural impulses passing over the osmoreceptors (see Figure 3–2). Intake or retention of fluid may cause extracellular fluid to be hypotonic. If extracellular fluid surrounding the osmoreceptor cells is hypotonic, water moves into the osmoreceptors and they swell. The neural impulses are slowed down as they pass over this larger cell surface area. The slowed neural impulses result in decreased ADH secretion. The decreased amount of ADH in the blood causes the distal tubules of the kidneys to reabsorb less water from the glomerular filtrate into the body. This process results in an increase in urinary output of a more dilute urine (see Figure 3–3).

Conversely, when fluid intake is decreased or body fluid is lost, the extracellular fluid becomes concentrated or hypertonic.

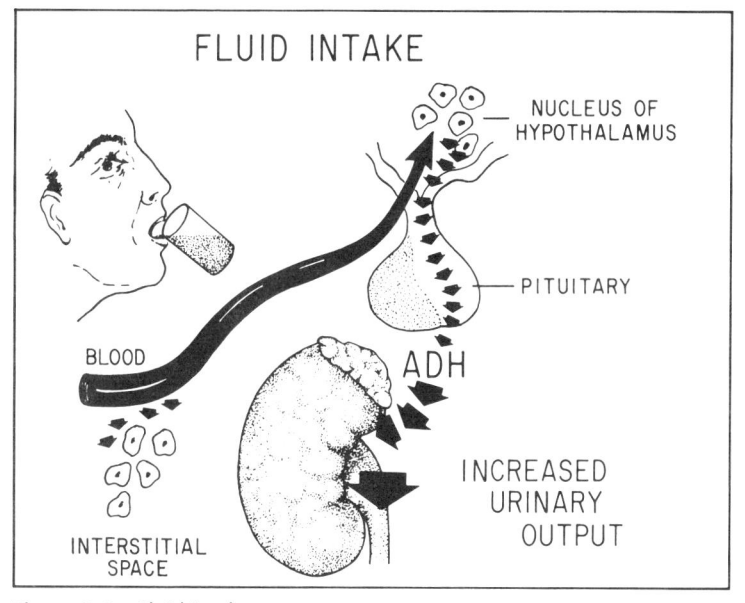

Figure 3–3 *Fluid intake.*

Water moves out of the osmoreceptor cells and they shrink. Neural impulses can now pass over the reduced surface area of the cell more rapidly, thus increasing the output of ADH (see Figure 3–2). The increased amounts of ADH in the blood act upon the loop of Henle in the kidney, increasing water reabsorption from the glomerular filtrate into the blood. The increased amount of water returns the tonicity of the extracellular fluid to equilibrium with that of the intracellular fluid. The result is a decrease in urinary output until osmotic equilibrium between intracellular and extracellular fluid is reached (see Figure 3–4).

Aldosterone, a hormone continuously secreted in small amounts by the adrenal cortex, acts upon the kidneys to influence renal control of body fluid levels of sodium and potassium (see Figure 3–5). As the cations sodium and potassium are retained or excreted, the anions such as chloride and bicarbonate are also

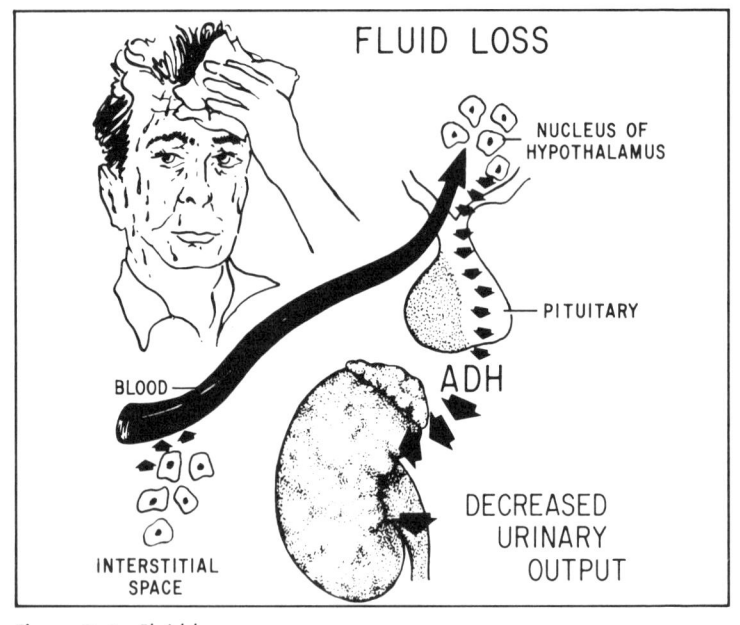

Figure 3–4 *Fluid loss.*

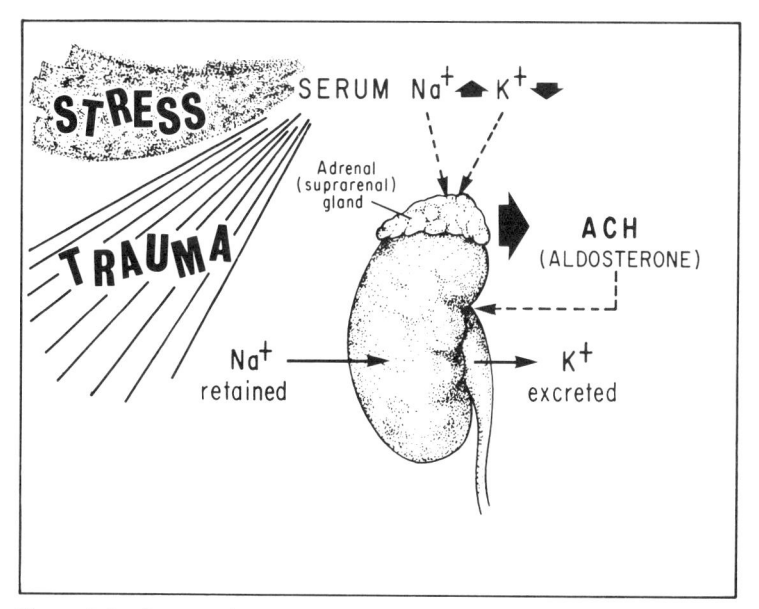

Figure 3-5 *Stress and trauma.*

retained or excreted respectively because of the electrical attraction between the oppositely charged cations and anions. The rate of secretion of aldosterone can be increased greatly by any one of or a combination of the following stimuli:

1. Reduced sodium concentration in body extracellular fluids
2. Reduced extracellular fluid volume
3. High extracellular concentrations of potassium
4. Physical or psychological stress such as fear, burns, trauma, surgery, and cardiac failure

Aldosterone acts on the kidneys to cause retention of sodium followed by water retention and accompanied by potassium excretion.[3]

[3] Arthur Guyton, *A Textbook of Medical Physiology,* 2d ed., W. B. Saunders Company, Philadelphia, 1961, pp. 99–100.

Blood volume changes affect urinary output. Increases in blood to the kidney, such as that accompanying physical exercise, causes increased urinary output; whereas a decreased renal blood volume, as in the case of hemorrhage, causes a decreased urinary output.

The effect of changes in blood volume on urinary output occur because (1) changes in blood volume affect the glomerular arterial pressure causing more or less glomerular filtrate to be formed, and (2) changes in blood volume affect secretion of ADH and aldosterone, which in turn controls water and sodium excretion respectively. Further, water is required to excrete sodium, and so sodium excretion or reabsorption also affects urinary output.

REGULATION OF ACID-BASE BALANCE

The body must maintain a concentration of hydrogen ions which is conducive to optimal cellular function. Slight changes in hydrogen ion concentrations in body fluid can cause acceleration or depression of the rate of chemical reactions taking place in the cells.

The term "pH" is used to express the hydrogen ion concentration of a fluid. A low arterial blood pH indicates a high hydrogen ion concentration, a state clinically referred to as *acidosis*. A high pH in arterial blood indicates a low hydrogen ion concentration, the clinical state known as *alkalosis*. The normal pH range for arterial blood is 7.35 to 7.45. An arterial blood pH of 7.0 is the lower limit of H^+ ion concentration compatible with life and the upper limit is a pH of 7.8.

The body has three simultaneously and constantly occurring mechanisms which regulate the acid-base balance of body fluids (see Figure 3–6) by altering, retaining, or excreting the hydrogen ions which are released during a variety or normal metabolic reactions.

Immediate regulation of H^+ ion concentration in body fluids is carried out by substances called *buffers*. Acid-base buffers are chemical compounds that prevent marked changes in hydrogen

BUFFERS

HCl + NaHCO$_3$ ⇌ NaCl + H$_2$CO$_3$

H$_2$O + CO$_2$

RESPIRATORY

H$_2$O + CO$_2$

RENAL

AMMONIA
HYDROGEN IONS

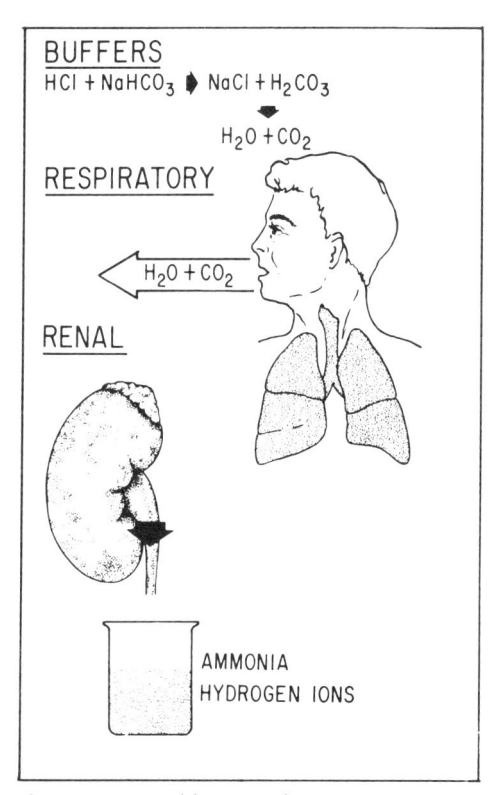

Figure 3–6 *Acid-base regulation.*

ion concentrations when acidic or basic substances are added to a solution. In the body there are four major buffer systems operating in the blood, kidneys, and cells. One of these four systems, the bicarbonate buffer system, if not the most powerful, is probably the most important because its chemical elements can be regulated by the lungs and kidneys.

The bicarbonate buffer system is composed of a mixture of carbonic acid (H$_2$CO$_3$) and a bicarbonate salt of sodium (NaHCO$_3$), potassium, calcium, or magnesium. When an acid or base is added to body fluid the bicarbonate buffer system functions in the following manner:

1. Addition of acid such as hydrochloric acid

$$HCl + NaHCO_3 \rightarrow H_2CO_3 + NaCl$$

2. Addition of base such as sodium hydroxide

$$NaOH + H_2CO_3 \rightarrow NaHCO_3 + H_2O$$

Carbonic acid is a weak acid which constantly breaks down and reforms into carbon dioxide and water ($H_2CO_3 \rightleftharpoons CO_2 + H_2O$) or hydrogen ions and bicarbonate ions ($H_2CO_3 \rightleftharpoons H^+ + HCO_3^-$).

The end products produced by the bicarbonate buffer system are readily excreted by the body. Carbon dioxide and water are excreted by the lungs, and the hydrogen ions or bicarbonate ions or both are excreted by the kidneys. The buffer systems function within a fraction of a second to prevent deviations in the pH of body fluids outside the normal ranges.

The second mechanism is the respiratory system, which acts as the backup system in regulation of the body's acid-base balance. When the normal blood levels of carbon dioxide are sufficiently altered, the respiratory centers of the brain are stimulated (by increases in carbon dioxide) or inhibited (by decreases in carbon dioxide) and, in turn, cause an increase or decrease of the rate and depth of respiration. This change in respiration favors the elimination or retention of carbon dioxide as necessary to return the blood levels of this substance to normal. The respiratory acid-base regulatory mechanism takes one to three minutes to be effective.

Renal regulation, the third mechanism, assumes the major role should the alterations in the acid-base balance of the body continue over long periods of time. Renal regulation also operates when acid-base alterations occur to a degree which cannot be corrected by the immediate and short-term responses of either the buffer systems or the respiratory system. The renal regulatory mechanism takes from several hours to one or more days to operate and acts by tubular excretion of hydrogen ions and ammonia into the urine.[4]

Some generalizations drawn from the foregoing discussions about the regulation of body fluid and electrolytes which may be of value to the nurse are as follows:

1. Urinary output of the patient is a critical indicator of the body's attempt to conserve or its need to excrete fluid or electrolytes or both.

2. Increases in urinary output are related to sodium excretion, so that sodium depletion may accompany copious urinary losses.

3. Intake of fluids affects the output of urine, and the two must be balanced for the patient to function normally.

4. Stress affects urinary output by initially causing retention of sodium and fluid. One expects decreased urinary output when the patient has undergone stress.

5. During stress, loss of potassium through the urine is increased above usual limits.

6. Any clinical state which changes blood volume to the kidney will affect urinary output of the patient (that is, vasodilation as a result of administration of medications or foods containing vasodilators, changes in blood pressure, congestive heart failure).

7. Changes in respiratory rate and depth not due to physical exertion may be indicative of or precipitate changes in the patient's acid-base balance.

8. Changes in the urinary pH, or urine having a strong ammonia odor, may be indicative of alteration of the patient's acid-base balance.

---

[4] Guyton, op cit., pp. 111–122.

FOUR
AVENUES OF GAINS AND LOSSES OF BODY FLUID AND ELECTROLYTES

Water is taken directly into the body by mouth or in food. One thousand gm of food can yield up to 1000 cc of metabolic water. As a general rule approximately 10 cc of water is produced by oxidation of 100 calories of fat, carbohydrate, or protein. A 1000-calorie diet yields 100 cc of water.

Were an individual to have no fluid intake at all, his body would continue to lose 1500 cc of fluid daily. This is called _obligatory fluid loss_. Obligatory fluid loss occurs in part from evaporation of water from the skin and in part from exhalation during respiration. These two avenues of loss are known as _insensible loss_. We normally lose between 900 and 1000 cc daily by these routes. The smallest amount of urine necessary for a normal kidney to excrete the waste products of a day's metabolism is 600 cc. Impaired kidney function increases the amount of urine (see Figure 4–1) necessary to excrete daily body wastes.[1] Thus, if the minimum daily obligatory fluid loss is 1500 cc, the minimum requirement for daily fluid intake, directly or in food, is 1500 cc (see Table 4–1). Losses through the kidneys and insensible losses may occur in excess of these minimum amounts. On a hot summer day we sweat profusely. Visible sweat over a course of 24 hours may approximate an additional loss of 1000 to 2000 cc. It is estimated that perspiration of a patient requiring a single change of bedclothes represents at least 1000 cc of water lost. The actual urinary output of an individual will vary considerably from the minimum of 600 cc depending upon fluid intake, the amount of metabolic wastes to be excreted, and how well the kidneys are functioning. Patients with stepped-up metabolic rates as in fever

[1] Stanley Mikal, *Homeostasis in Man*, Little, Brown and Company, Boston, 1967, pp. 4–5.

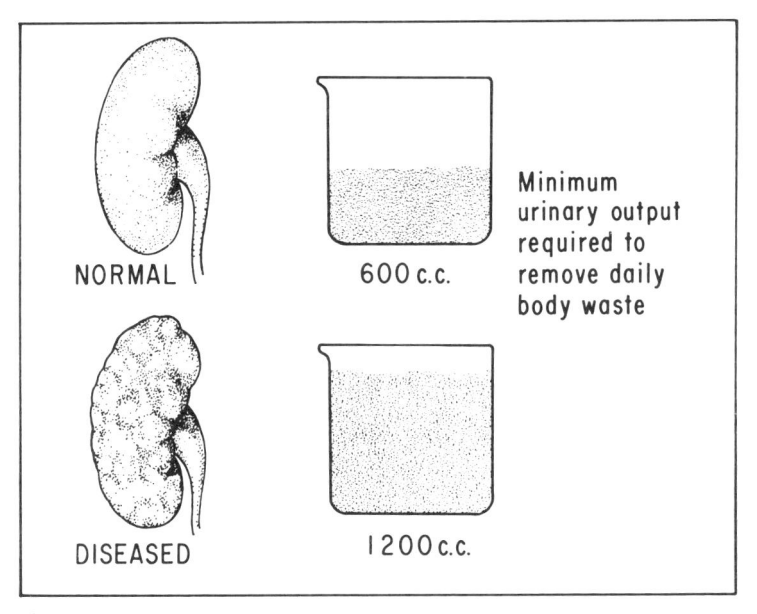

Figure 4–1 *Minimum urinary output.*

Table 4–1 *Fluid and Electrolyte Loss and Replacement in Adults*

Type of loss	Amount lost (per 24 hr)	Replacement required (per 24 hr)
Obligatory fluid		
Insensible: sweat, respiration	900–1000 cc	900–1500 cc
Urine	600–1500 cc	600–1500 cc
Feces	100 cc	Usually replaced by oxidation of nutrients
Sodium	4 gm	Usually replaced by normal diet
Potassium	2–3 gm	Usually replaced by normal diet

Source: Harry Statland, *Fluid and Electrolytes in Practice*, 2d ed., J. B. Lippincott Company, Philadelphia, 1957; also Stanley Mikal, *Homeostasis in Man*, Little, Brown and Company, Boston, 1967.

or thyrotoxicosis may have increased urinary outputs. Intake of fluid must be adequate to replace continuous fluid losses or the fluid will be drawn from the tissues and cells.

Patients who are not eating have almost the same water requirements for excretion of wastes as those who are eating. The reason for this is that the fasting patient has increased protein and fat breakdown because these nutrients are converted to carbohydrates for energy. The end waste products of protein and fat catabolism require water to be excreted by the kidneys. Patients receiving high protein diets or tube feedings also lose fluid excreting the protein catabolic waste.

Potassium is consumed in sufficient quantities in the average diet to replace daily losses of this cation from the kidney. If potassium intake is reduced, the kidneys continue to lose potassium and depletion can soon occur. On the other hand, daily potassium loss may increase under certain conditions. Potassium content of sweat, for example, is ordinarily low, but visible perspiration may contain up to 75 mEq of potassium per liter of sweat, thus increasing the need for replacement. Potassium deficiency may also be associated with vomiting and diarrhea.

Sodium intake in the usual diet is sufficient to supply body needs. When sodium intake is decreased or stopped, the kidney decreases its output of sodium in the urine. Thus, if there are no other routes of loss, the body can get along for quite a while with decreased sodium intake. Visible perspiration can lead to salt deficits, especially in individuals losing additional sodium by abnormal routes.

Water lost in feces usually approximates the water gained from the oxidation of carbohydrates, fats, and proteins unless the patient's output of feces is increased, as in diarrhea. Thus, normally, water loss by defecation in effect is negligible.

Hydrogen ions, the "acid" ions, are taken in by mouth (in negligible amounts) and are also generated by the oxidation of food and tissue. In this latter instance, the end products of combustion of carbohydrates, fats, and proteins produce carbon dioxide which is continuously combining with water to form carbonic acid. This acid, in turn, may then dissociate back into carbon dioxide and water or into hydrogen ions and bicarbonate ions (see Chapter 3). In addition to carbon dioxide other acid substances are formed during body metabolism.

Bicarbonate ions, the "base" ions, are primarily formed from the dissociation of carbonic acid into hydrogen ions and bicarbonate ions.[2]

Normally hydrogen and bicarbonate ions are excreted through respiratory or renal excretion as described earlier.

Certain clinical states, including measures designed to be therapeutic, may also result in alterations in fluid and electrolyte gain or loss from the body.

CLINICAL STATES AFFECTING FLUID AND ELECTROLYTE BALANCE

Clinical states which alter fluid and electrolyte balance may be classified into six groups (see Table 4–2). The first classification includes those states which precipitate and accentuate the normal

[2] Douglas A. K. Black, *Essentials of Fluid Balance*, 4th ed., Blackwell Scientific Publications, Ltd., Oxford, 1967, pp. 108–109.

Table 4–2 *Classification of Common Clinical States Affecting Fluid and Electrolyte Balance*

Clinical state	Effect on fluid and electrolyte balance
Pain Anesthesia Fear Trauma	Heightened response to stress
Renal failure Pulmonary emphysema Pituitary tumors Adrenocortical destruction	Impaired acid-base regulatory mechanism
Congestive heart failure Blood loss Immobilization	Impaired fluid circulation
Sweating Diarrhea Increased urinary output Increased electrolyte output in urine	Excessive loss of fluid by normal routes
"-ostomies" Nasogastric suction Bleeding "-centeses" Vomiting	Excessive loss of fluid by abnormal routes
Tube feedings of concentrated solutes Parenteral infusions administered incorrectly Infant feedings of insufficiently diluted cow's milk	Increased fluid and electrolytes

stress responses of the body. The stress response, resulting from increased aldosterone secretion, normally includes decreased urinary output, retention of sodium accompanied by excretion of potassium, and changes in circulating blood volume. In addition, perspiration and respirations are increased under stress. Pain, fear, trauma of surgery, and anesthesia are all examples of clinical states which accentuate or prolong normal stress responses. As a result patients under stress retain sodium and water, lose potassium, and lose fluid by perspiration and respirations, and shifts in fluid occur decreasing circulating blood volume. The resulting fluid and electrolyte imbalance must be corrected. Extrinsic trauma such as burns or massive crushing injuries precipitates and accentuates the normal body response to stress but also results in actual loss of large amounts of fluid, internal fluid shifts, and electrolyte changes which occur in response to the decreased extracellular fluid volume and physical stress. Shock and death may result from any of these clinical states if fluid and electrolyte imbalances are not promptly corrected.

Sometimes the regulatory mechanisms of the kidney, respiration, adrenocortical steroids, or pituitary hormones, which usually maintain fluid and electrolyte balance, may become defective. Here, the patient may experience excessive retention or loss of electrolytes and fluid depending upon the defective mechanism and the extent of the pathological process. A common clinical state which falls in this second category is renal failure.

The third category is that of clinical states due to defects of body fluid circulation such as congestive heart failure, in which case the patient retains fluid in the tissues while experiencing a decrease in circulating blood volume. The patient may experience defects of circulation due to loss of blood from trauma or fluid shifts due to immobilization. The end result is decreased circulating blood volume.

The fourth and fifth categories, excessive loss of fluids and electrolytes by normal and abnormal routes, are of special interest to nurses since many of the clinical states so classified are commonly encountered. In addition, the prevention of the occurrence of these clinical states is possible and within the realm of independent nurse action during the care of patients. Examples of excessive loss of fluid by normal routes include sweating, diarrhea, salivary drainage, and urinary loss or electrolyte loss as a result of drug effects. Excessive loss of fluid by abnormal routes includes vomiting, drainage from ileostomies, colostomies, cecostomies, fistulas, wounds, and gastrointestinal suction and irrigation, and the removal of fluid by thoracentesis or paracentesis. You will note in Tables 4-3 and 4-4 the ranges of electrolyte composition of gastrointestinal secretions as well as of urine and sweat.

Table 4-3 *Electrolyte Composition of Gastrointestinal Secretions and Excretions*

Intestinal tract locality	Na^+ (mEq/liter)*	K^+ (mEq/liter)*	Cl^- (mEq/liter)*	HCO_3^- (mEq/liter)*
Saliva	9	25.8	10	(12–18)†
Gastric juice (fasting)	60 (10–115)	10 (1.0–35)	85 (8–150)	(0–15)
Pancreatic fistula	141 (115–150)	4.6 (2.5–7.5)	76.0 (55–95)	121
Biliary tract fistula	148 (130–160)	5.0 (2.8–12)	101 (90–118)	40
Jejunal suction (small bowel secretion)	111 (85–150)	4.6 (2.3–8.0)	104 (45–125)	31
Ileum suction	117 (85–118)	5.0 (2.5–8.0)	105.0 (60–127)	
Ileostomy (recent)	129 (106–143)	11.0 (6–29)	116 (90–136)	
Ileostomy (old)	46	3.0	21.4	
Cecostomy	79 (45–135)	20 (5–45)	45 (18–88)	
Stools—Children Normal Very diarrheal	1.8* 11.6*	3.8* 17.5*	0.6* 8.0*	

* Values given in milliequivalents per 24 hours.
† Values in parentheses represent ranges.
Source: John Bland, *Clinical Metabolism of Body Water and Electrolytes,* W. B. Saunders Company, Philadelphia, 1963.

Table 4–4 *Electrolyte Composition of Urine and Sweat*

Substance	Urine	Sweat
Na	128 mEq./liter	80 mEq.
K	60	5
Ca	4.8	1
Mg	15	0.5
Cl	134	86.5
Urea-N	18.2 mg.%	15 mg.%
Glucose	0	2
Lactic acid	—	35
Protein	—	0 gm.%

Source: Arthur Guyton, *Textbook of Medical Physiology,* 2nd edition. W.B. Saunders Company, Philadelphia, 1961, pp. 92, 955.

FIVE
BODY RESPONSES TO CHANGES IN BODY FLUID, ELECTROLYTES, AND ACID-BASE BALANCE

HOMEOSTASIS

The human organism presents to the observer a fascinating, awe-inspiring series of phenomena which enable the body to continue in a living state. During life the organism is constantly dynamic. The end result of the constant physiological changes taking place is the maintenance of the organism with a stable internal environment and the ability to continuously adapt to external environmental stressors. This condition of being, that is, constantly changing to maintain internal stability and to adapt externally, is *homeostasis*. The body has certain mechanisms by which it maintains homeostasis. These mechanisms occur in response to neurohormonal stimuli, which in turn have been elicited by some change in the internal or external milieu.

The normal fluid and electrolyte changes physiologically occurring in the internal milieu are regulated by the renal and respiratory mechanisms as well as the acid-base buffer systems as described in earlier chapters.

Unusual stressors affecting the internal or external milieu call forth a systemic response commonly known as the *stress response*. The stress response includes certain consistently appearing, identifiable, physiological reactions. These reactions include renal, respiratory, metabolic, sympathetic, and circulatory responses to neurohormonal stimulation. The stress response includes three stages: (1) alarm reaction, (2) adaptation or countershock reaction, (3) exhaustion. The former two stages are most intimately involved in the precipitation of fluid and electrolyte changes which may return the organism to a state of equilibrium. However, the same changes, in and of themselves and in the presence of continuing stress, may cause death if they are not corrected by medical therapy.

The alarm reaction is adrenergic; that is, its effects are the result of the secretion of the adrenergic hormones epinephrine and norepinephrine (see Figure 5–1). Epinephrine and norepinephrine cause vasoconstriction of visceral and cerebral blood vessels and muscular perfusion. In addition, a resulting decreased circulating blood volume leads to oliguria and acts as an added stimulus to the adrenal cortex to secrete the mineralocorticoids.

The second stage, or adaptation reaction, follows the alarm reaction in attempting to correct the homeostatic disequilibrium of the organism with the environment. This reaction is corticoid in nature, that is, is controlled by adrenal cortical secretions of mineralocorticoids, glucocorticoids, and androgens. The mineralocorticoid response of the adaptation reaction primarily affects fluid and electrolyte balance. It is stimulated by the pituitary adrenocorticotrophic hormone secretion, extracellular fluid volume (which is altered during the alarm stage), and serum concentrations of sodium and potassium.[1,2]

The resulting clinical manifestations are oliguria, weight gain, metabolic alkalosis, and potassium depletion.

[1] Guyton, op. cit., pp. 259–270, 987–988, 999–1001.
[2] Mikal, op. cit., pp. 93–98.

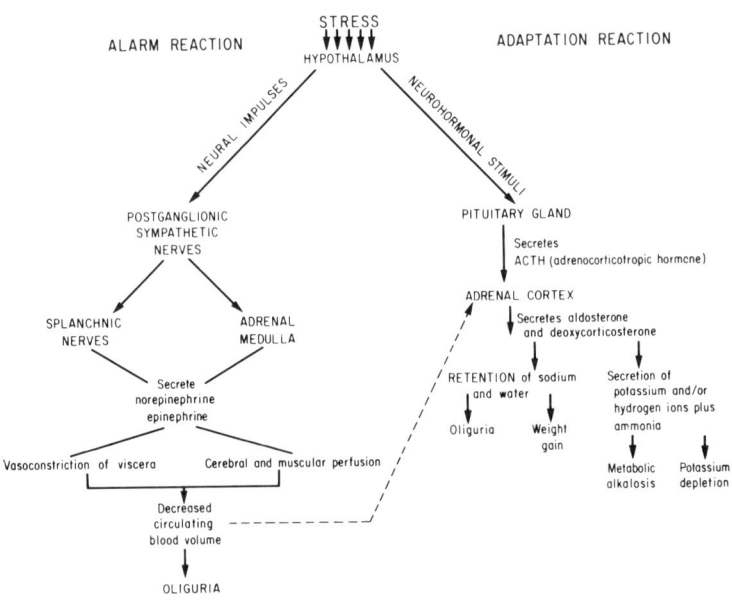

Figure 5-1 *Alterations in fluid and electrolytes due to stress response.*

Knowledge of the various physiological responses to alterations in the internal and external milieu facilitates prediction of fluid and electrolyte changes which will occur in association with certain clinical states. Prediction or recognition of the clinical manifestations accompanying changes in fluid and electrolyte balance is also possible when the nurse not only possesses but is able to use this knowledge.

BODY RESPONSES TO CHANGES IN BODY FLUID

Increased body fluid is accompanied by increased urination if renal function is not impaired. Slow increases in body fluid are accompanied by edema of extremities and periorbital edema (see Figure 5-2). Increases in body fluid in the presence of impaired renal function or increases in body fluid too rapid to be accom-

BODY WATER INCREASED

SLOW

PERIORBITAL EDEMA

DYSPNEA GURGLING RALES

EDEMA OF EXTREMITIES

RAPID

MENTAL IRRITABILITY

DYSPNEA GURGLING RALES

CONVULSIONS

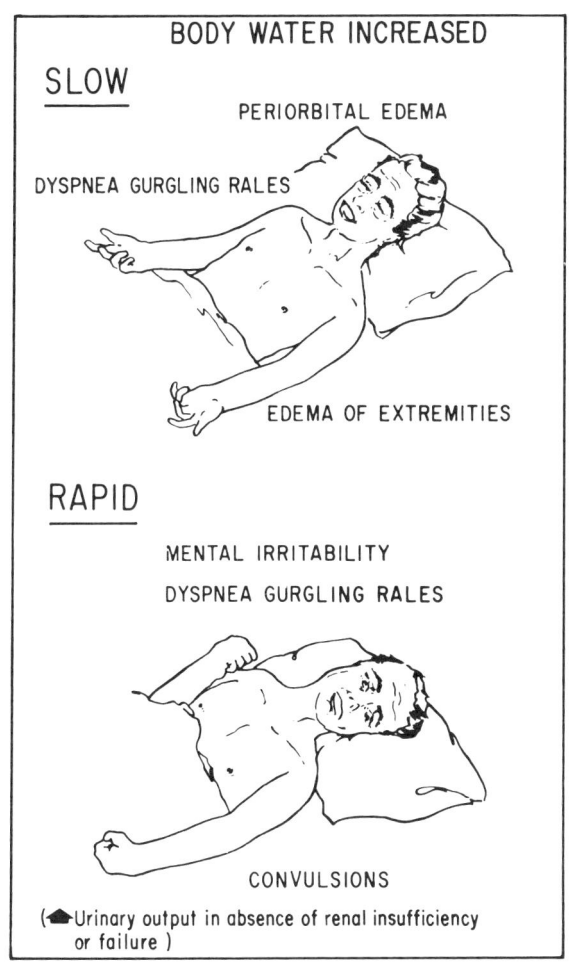

(⬅Urinary output in absence of renal insufficiency or failure)

Figure 5-2 *Body water increased.*

modated by normal kidney function result in signs of increased intracellular fluid in the brain, that is, mental irritability or convulsions or both. This is particularly true when these signs occur within 48 hours after surgery.[3] In patients with real or potential cardiac dysfunction there may also be signs of inability of the heart to assume the workload of circulating the increased fluid, that is, pulmonary edema, which may precede or accompany signs of increased fluid in the brain. The early symptoms of pulmonary edema include dyspnea and gurgling rales.

Signs of decreased body fluid are somewhat different for rapid loss than for slow loss. However, prolonged slow losses which are not corrected result ultimately in the same body responses as those for rapid fluid loss. The rapid loss of fluid may be real, as in hemorrhage, or relative, as in sudden fluid shifts from circulating blood volume to the interstitial spaces. Whether the losses are real or relative, the ultimate body responses are the same.

Slow fluid loss is accompanied by oliguria, thirst, elevated temperature, poor skin turgor, dry mucous membranes, and flushed, dry skin in the early stages (see Figure 5–3). In later stages

[3] Black, op. cit., pp. 34–36.

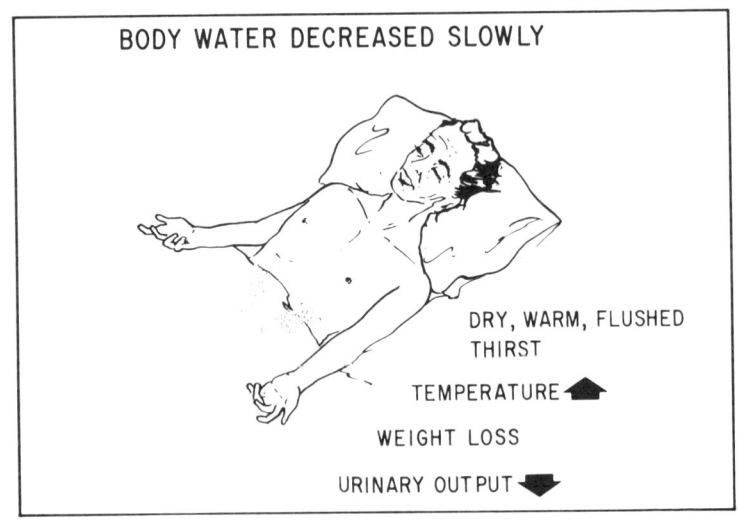

Figure 5–3 *Body water decreased slowly.*

of slow fluid loss, as well as in rapid fluid loss, the patient has extreme thirst, hypotension, restlessness and apprehension, oliguria which progresses to anuria, cold extremities, and pale or cyanotic, clammy skin (see Figure 5–4). If fluid loss is not corrected, the patient loses consciousness and dies. These symptoms, which precede the final stage of death, are recognizable as those of *shock*. Decreased oxygenation of tissue due to decreased circulating blood volume leads to cellular reactions which release large amounts of lactic acid. The accumulation of this acid places the patient in metabolic acidosis. If the acidosis is not relieved and circulation and oxygenation restored, irreversible cell damage and cell death occur. The end result of shock is a breakdown in homeostatic mechanisms and finally death of the patient. To recapitulate: slow fluid loss, if prolonged, leads to the same abnormal circumstances that produce shock as rapid fluid loss.[4]

[4] F. A. Simeone, "Shock—Its Nature and Treatment," *American Journal of Nursing,* 66(6): 1288–1289, 1966.

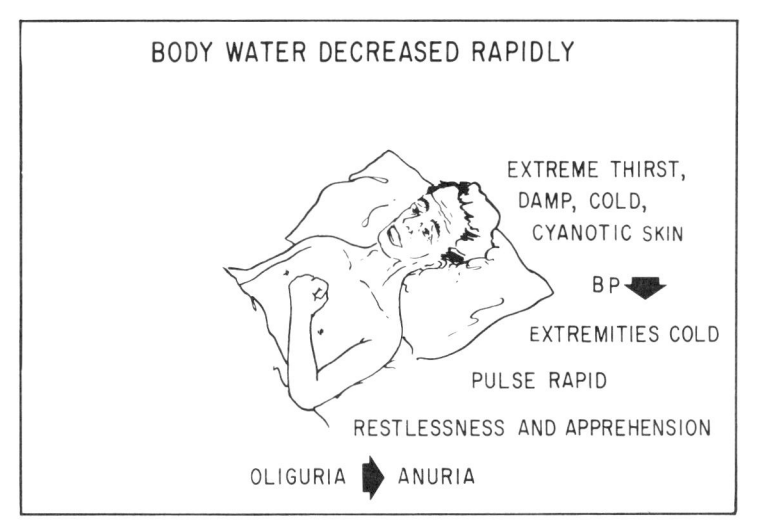

Figure 5–4 *Body water decreased rapidly.*

BODY RESPONSES TO CHANGES IN MAJOR ELECTROLYTES

Changes in fluid volume are usually accompanied by changes in the major electrolytes, sodium and potassium. Loss of fluid volume, particularly through gastrointestinal secretions, urine, or sweat, is usually accompanied by sodium depletion. Thus, sodium depletion (hyponatremia) (see Figure 5–5) is characterized by most of the symptoms for fluid loss especially those of rapid or prolonged fluid loss. Slowly developing sodium depletion is marked by abdominal cramps, weakness, and fatigue and progresses to the more serious shock-like symptoms if not corrected.

When potassium is abnormally lost from the body or is not taken in sufficient quantities to replace normal daily losses, abdominal distention may develop from softening of the smooth muscles of the intestines. Striated muscles also become soft as a result of cellular breakdown. The patient is weak. There is also a weak, rapid, irregular pulse and an increasing sensitivity of heart

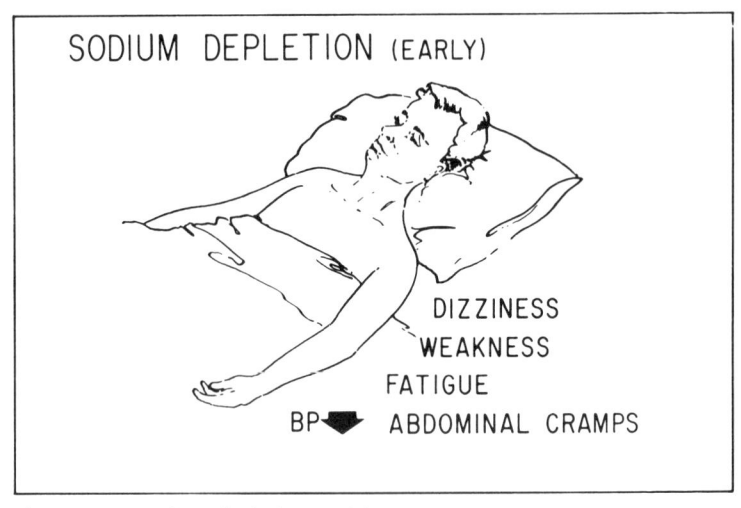

Figure 5–5 *Sodium depletion (early).*

muscle to digitalis and its derivatives. When decreased serum potassium (hypokalemia) develops, symptoms of digitalis toxicity may occur in patients receiving what are ordinarily considered to be therapeutic dosages of digitalis. The major symptom of digitalis toxicity is the development of cardiac arrhythmias. One is particularly alert for the onset of arrhythmic pulse in the digitalized cardiac patient receiving either thiazide or mercurial diuretics, since large amounts of potassium are lost with the diuresis. The end result of uncorrected potassium deficiency on heart muscle is heart block and death. Respiratory muscles may also become weak resulting in dyspnea in the potassium depleted patient. If the potassium depletion in patients with respiratory muscle involvement is not corrected, respiratory failure will result in death (see Figure 5–6).

When potassium is retained (see Figure 5–7) or increased in the body above normal levels (hyperkalemia), the patient experiences changes in sensation and exhibits behavioral changes. His pulse may be arrhythmic and slowed down. The patient may com-

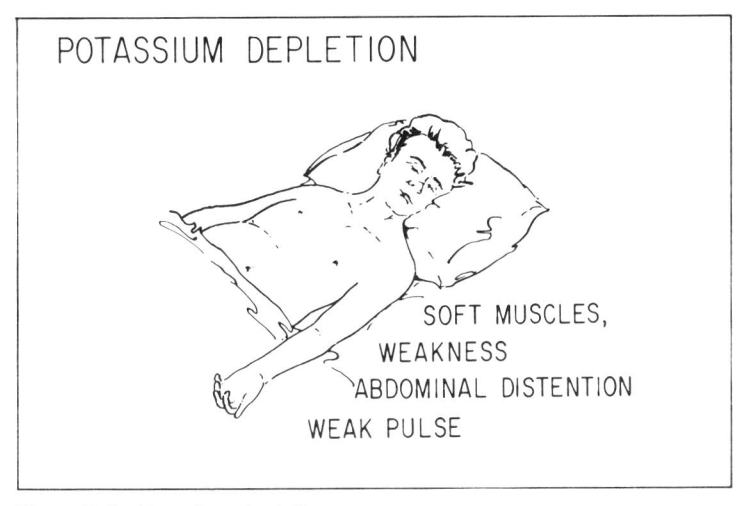

Figure 5–6 *Potassium depletion.*

POTASSIUM RETENTION

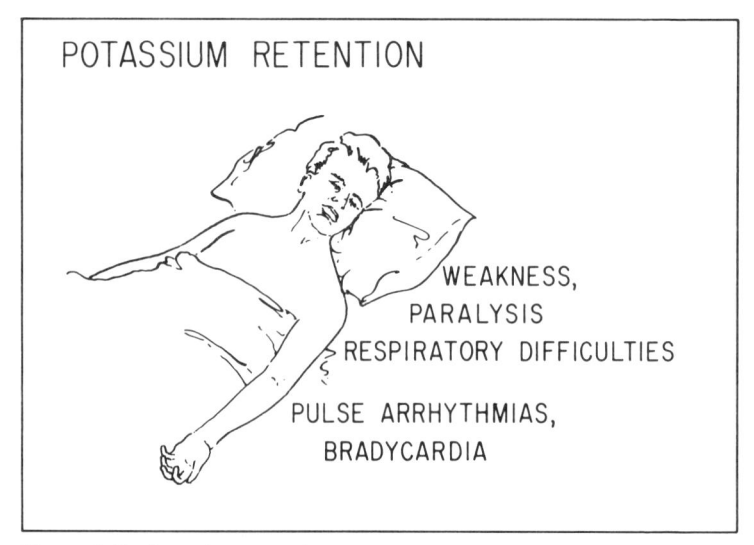

WEAKNESS,
PARALYSIS
RESPIRATORY DIFFICULTIES

PULSE ARRHYTHMIAS,
BRADYCARDIA

Figure 5-7 *Potassium retention.*

plain of tingling fingers and toes or of abdominal cramps. He may be restless and irritable. He may experience paresthesia of the scalp. Changes in myocardial conduction of nerve impulses may also be present. If the hyperkalemic condition is not corrected, muscles become weak and flaccid paralysis may develop. As mentioned earlier, when paralysis involves respiratory muscles, death may ensue. Cardiac arrest may also occur, causing death.[5,6]

Excessive retention of calcium (hypercalcemia) is commonly encountered in the patient with kidney disease and may result in deep bony pain and relaxed muscles. Calcium deficit (hypocalcemia) may develop as a concomitant to therapy to correct acidosis. Tingling fingers, tetany progressing to carpopedal spasm, and convulsions are characteristic symptoms of hypocalcemia.

The body response to other electrolyte excesses or deficits

---

[5] Guyton, op. cit., pp. 287–288.
[6] Black, op. cit., pp. 89–104.

usually occurs in conjunction with the responses to the major electrolyte imbalances and as such may be masked.

BODY RESPONSES TO ACID-BASE CHANGES

Changes in the acid-base balance of the body produce specific responses in addition to symptoms of the associated fluid and electrolyte state. Metabolic acidosis, a state in which there is an actual loss of base bicarbonate from extracellular fluid, produces deep, rapid respiration; the patient may be disoriented. There is a strong ammonia-like odor to the urine. The change in respiration occurs as a physiological compensatory mechanism to get rid of carbon dioxide and to move the patient toward acid-base balance. Diarrhea, vomiting, uremia, and diabetes mellitus are all common causes of metabolic acidosis.

Metabolic alkalosis, that is, an increase in base bicarbonate, is accompanied by depressed respirations, hypertonic muscles, tetany, and alkaline urine. Alkalosis is not as common as acidosis and usually does not occur spontaneously but arises from the imposition of alkali loads, for example, excessive ingestion of alkaline drugs like sodium bicarbonate or antacids.

Acidosis or alkalosis due to increased or inhibited respirations may also develop; however, the symptoms which the nurse may observe are similar to those of metabolically caused acidosis or alkalosis. The important point to remember here is that a patient having respiratory changes such as increased respiratory rate due to fever or hysteria may develop alkalosis, whereas decreased respiration in a patient with pneumonia or emphysema may lead to acidosis. If the imbalances are not corrected the patient may die.

PART TWO
NURSING INTERVENTION IN
MAINTENANCE AND RESTORATION
OF FLUID AND ELECTROLYTE BALANCE

SIX
THE NURSE'S ROLE IN OBSERVATION AND ASSESSMENT

OBSERVATION

The nurse's role in the maintenance and restoration of fluid and electrolyte balance rests in her ability to know when to observe, what to observe, and how to assess her observations.

The nurse who is aware of the enormous variety of clinical states which may result in changes in fluid and electrolytes also recognizes that continual vigilance is required in this respect for all patients. The astute nurse does not dismiss any patient complaint until she has assessed it in the light of the information on the patient's chart and her personal observation through interaction with the patient. She anticipates and is alert for the onset of symptoms of fluid and electrolyte imbalance in certain patients, such as the vomiting patient or the one with diarrhea.

What does the nurse observe about the patient? These observations may be categorized into easily recalled classifications as follows (see Table 6–1 and Figure 6–1).

Physical Appearance and Activity

The nurse observes the patient's skin for changes in color, temperature, turgor, and moisture. Is the patient pale, cyanosed, or flushed? Perhaps he has patches of reddened areas on his face or body. Is the skin cold or warm to the touch? Is the patient's skin damp, wet, or dry? If visible sweat is present, how long has it persisted? Does the skin have elasticity? The mucous membranes and nail beds should also be observed for color changes. Pressure on nail beds may reveal slow return of color. Capillary filling slows when changes are taking place in circulating blood volume as may occur during severe dehydration, sodium depletion, and other clinical states described in Chapter 5. Mucous membranes may be dry and the patient may complain of thirst when rapid or slow loss of body fluid is in progress.

Frequently, the level of the patient's activity may be an early

Table 6–1 *Observation and Assessment Aids*

Source	Observation by nurse
Patient	Physical appearance Activity Sensory status Vital signs Gastrointestinal output Urinary output Daily weight
Chart	Diagnosis Treatment Medication Previous health Laboratory reports Intake and output

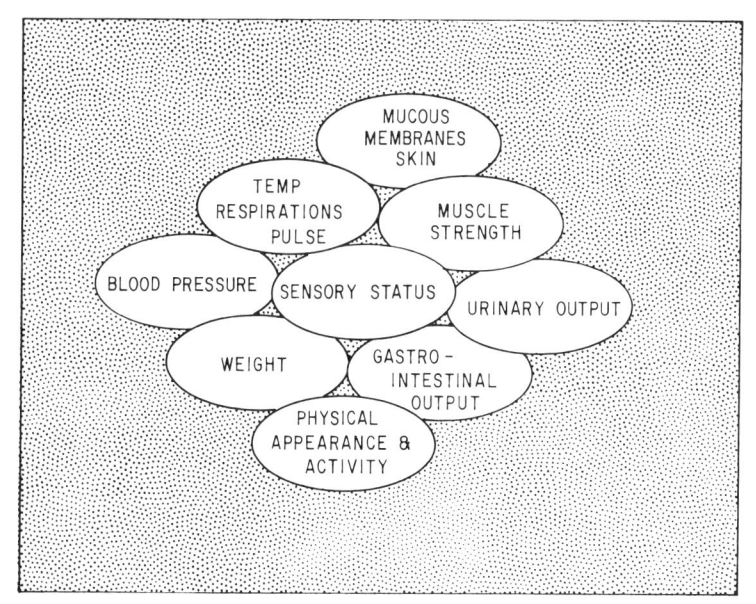

Figure 6–1 *Observations.*

indicator of associated fluid or electrolyte imbalances. Restlessness or visible signs of apprehension may accompany early loss of extracellular fluid. Clinical states such as hemorrhage, neurogenic or vasogenic reactions which may accompany trauma or follow anesthesia, or overwhelming infections may also be precipitating factors in extracellular fluid loss.

Electrolyte losses of potassium or sodium as well as retention of potassium or calcium are accompanied by changes in neuromuscular irritability. The nurse may observe the patient to be extremely fatigued, weak, anorectic, or lethargic. The weakness may be as slight as diminished gripping power or as extensive as flaccid paralysis of the skeletal muscles.

The patient may complain of abdominal cramps when he is losing sodium. Abdominal distention due to loss of tone of the smooth muscle in intestinal walls may be an early indication of potassium depletion. The nurse should be particularly observant for signs of potassium depletion in patients who have undergone surgery, since sodium retention and potassium excretion are concomitants of the body's response to physiological stress. The belly portion of the large muscles in the arms and legs may become soft and mushy as a result of loss of potassium.

The nurse observes the soft tissues over the sacrum, of the extremities, and surrounding the eyes for signs of fluid retention (edema). Such retention may accompany clinical states in which fluid intake increases beyond the patient's renal limits for excretion or in which there is increased sodium retention.

Muscle twitching should be anticipated in patients who may potentially lose calcium, such as occurs in nephrotic children receiving sodium exchange resins over a long period of time. Contraction of smooth muscle in patients with low serum calcium may also produce abdominal cramps, whereas muscular fasciculations, tremors, and choreiform movements may be observed when there is a loss of magnesium. Since gastric juice is high in magnesium, the nurse should be alert for signs of magnesium loss when patients have been vomiting or have undergone prolonged gastric suction.[1, 2, 3]

In general, we can say that signs of changes in neuromuscular irritability should alert the nurse to the possibility of electrolyte derangement.

Sensory Status

The nurse evaluates the patient's sensory status in terms of irritability, orientation to time, place, and person, degrees of confusion, and apathy. Mental irritability may be an early indication of shifts of fluid from the extracellular to the intracellular space and should be particularly noted during the administration of

[1] Mikal, op. cit., pp. 32–45, 407–415, 423–427.
[2] Statland, op. cit., p. 135.
[3] Black, op. cit., pp. 39–104.

parenteral fluids. Forgetfulness can be an early sign of tissue hypoxia. The patient's sensory status is also affected by loss of calcium, increases in magnesium, and retention or loss of potassium. Numbness and tingling of extremities may be observed in retention of potassium.

Vital Signs

Too frequently, observation of the patient's vital signs becomes routine rather than astute. Knowledgeable observation of these signs is requisite to the kind of judgment and intervention that characterizes intelligent nursing care.

Temperature elevations occur concomitantly with early water depletion. The nurse should be aware not only that the onset of a temperature elevation may signal previous water loss but that the present elevation may increase the rate at which further water loss will occur. A falling body temperature, particularly following periods of temperature elevation, may be an indication not of improvement in the patient's status but of the onset of fluid shifts of a serious nature.

Pulse rate changes occur in relation to changes in potassium balance, sodium depletion, and fluid shifts which affect the circulating blood volume. In the last two instances, tachycardia may be observed but is not an inevitable concomitant. For example, an aged person with some degree of heart block may show little change in pulse rate despite conditions of circulatory failure.[4] Arrhythmic pulse rates should be noted particularly in patients who might potentially retain or excrete potassium.

Observations of the patient's respiratory rate, depth, and volume are important in evaluating the effectiveness of the respiratory acid-base regulatory mechanism. Ordinarily the nurse is alert for changes in rate and depth of respiration. However, under specific circumstances she may also have to measure the minute ventilation of the patient's respirations (that is, patients in or prone

[4] Simeone, op. cit., pp. 1287–1288.

to manifest acute respiratory failure and associated respiratory acidosis).[5]

The observation of the immobilized patient's respirations is of prime importance in preventing oxygen-carbon dioxide imbalance, respiratory acidosis, and possibly death. In addition to the patient's respiratory rate, depth, and volume, the nurse considers the quality of the patient's respiration in terms of whether it is wet or dry, easy or labored. She also watches to see if the patient uses his neck muscles or abdominal muscles in breathing.[6]

Blood pressure changes are primarily associated with conditions in which the fluid in the vascular compartment is compromised. Generally speaking, blood pressure falls in association with loss of circulating blood volume for whatever reason—sodium and water depletion, fluid shifts in the body, blood loss, and so forth. The nurse should be alert for two additional observations in relation to blood pressure. First, she should note not only the blood pressure but also the pulse pressure. When blood pressure changes are due to blood loss, the systolic pressure falls more rapidly than the diastolic pressure so that the pulse pressure falls (systolic pressure minus diastolic pressure equals pulse pressure). A patient whose blood pressure is falling because of blood loss needs more immediate therapy than one whose pressure is falling because of plasma volume shifts due to immobilization.

Occasionally, as a result of the initial response of the body to stress, the blood pressure may be normal or even above normal following a serious injury or blood loss. During the initial response, release of hormones by the adrenals and sympathetic nerve endings causes an initial vasoconstriction of "low priority" organs such as the kidneys, skin, and viscera. The blood thus shunted assists in maintaining circulating blood volume and in cerebral and muscular tissue perfusion. Patients under stress should be closely observed and supported since the addition of

[5] Louise Nett and Thomas Petty, "Acute Respiratory Failure," *American Journal of Nursing,* 67(9): 1848, 1967.
[6] Edith Olsen et al., "The Hazards of Immobility," *American Journal of Nursing,* 67(4): 784, 1967.

minor physical stress such as a change of position may tip the scale from compensated maintenance of circulating blood volume to decompensation, further derangement of metabolic processes, and death.[7, 8]

Observation of blood pressure in association with decreased urinary output is of critical importance in determining the type of fluid replacement needed by the patient whose fluid balance is deranged by burns. A falling blood pressure indicates the need for more colloid to hold fluid intravascularly; a normal blood pressure signals the need for additional electrolytes or water.[9, 10]

Gastrointestinal Output

In her observation of gastrointestinal output, the nurse must be alert to five basic factors:

1. Source
2. Amount
3. Frequency
4. Color
5. Consistency

A review of Table 4–3 (see p. 40) indicates not only a variety of potential sources of gastrointestinal output but also their relative electrolytic components. In addition to observing for the more obvious losses such as gastrointestinal suction, vomiting, diarrhea, fistula drainage, "-ostomies," and paracentesis drainages, the nurse should be aware of covert modes of gastrointestinal output. Purgatives and enemas used preoperatively or before treatment of the gastrointestinal tract deplete the patient of water, potassium, calcium, magnesium, and phosphorus. There should be close obser-

---

[7] Simeone, loc. cit.
[8] Mikal, op. cit., pp. 93–95.
[9] Duane Larson and Rita Gaston, "Current Trends in the Care of Burned Patients," *American Journal of Nursing*, 67(2): 322, 1967.
[10] Mikal, op. cit., pp. 307–309.

vation of the amount of fluid returned by enemas as well as that excreted as a result of laxatives, and evaluation should be made in the light of the patient's intake and other factors to be discussed later under Assessment.[11, 12]

Urinary Output

Urinary output is of paramount significance in the evaluation of the patient's fluid and electrolyte balance. The amount of output is indicative of renal water excretory function or the amount of extracellular water circulating in the vascular space. The chemistry of the urine is indicative of renal regulation of electrolytic constituents of the body fluid, whereas the physical characteristics of urine (that is, odor, color, and specific gravity) are primarily indicative of the concentrating and diluting powers of the kidney. The nurse must observe not only the amount of urine voided by the patient but its odor, color, and frequency. In certain instances the specific gravity will also be measured on the unit. Generally, however, the nurse will need to refer to the laboratory urinalysis report for additional information such as specific gravity, urine casts, and red blood cells. Prior to surgery the urinary status of the patient is closely observed by the nurse, who, in turn, relays any information which will assist the doctor in anticipating problems of fluid and electrolyte balance.

During the first few days of the postoperative period, the nurse expects the patient to exhibit a decreased urinary output having a maximal period of decreased output within the 24 hours immediately after surgery. The output then returns to a normal level after 72 hours.[13, 14]

Any clinical state which changes the circulating blood vol-

[11] M. F. Dunning and F. Pleem, "Potassium Depletion by Enemas," *American Journal of Medicine*, 20: 789–792, May, 1956.
[12] Mikal, op. cit., pp. 387–394.
[13] Mikal, op. cit., pp. 401–404.
[14] June Abbey, "Nursing Observations of Fluid Imbalance," *Nursing Clinics of North America*, 3(1): 79, 1968.

ume will alter urinary output. The nurse is alert for the expected change and recognizes and reports not only the change, should it occur, but deviations from expected values as they arise.

Daily Weight

Daily weighing of the patient is one of the most valuable methods for determining his fluid and metabolic change. It is important therefore to weigh the patient accurately on admission to serve as a base-line measurement.

The surgical patient is expected to demonstrate early weight gain indicative of normal postoperative fluid retention, whereas loss of 1.1 pound or more per day for two days postoperatively suggests dehydration. Subsequently, a loss of weight may occur as a result of the tissue oxidation due to the body's response to stress. Postoperative weight has little significance if the weight of drainage tubes, bedclothing, and clamps is not taken into account. Nasogastric tubes weigh approximately one ounce, and Kelly clamps weigh as much as three to four ounces. Together these weights mask one-fourth of the anticipated weight loss for the first postoperative day. Conditions for weighing should be as uniform as possible, taking place at the same time of day and on the same scale.[15, 16, 17]

Close observation of the patient's daily weight is important in a variety of medical conditions in which fluid loss or gain must be monitored as a guide to adequate replacement or diuresis. Weight is of particular significance in respect to fluid balance for the patient with chronic renal failure, congestive heart failure, or ulcerative colitis, or patients on chronic dialysis. When she is weighing the hospitalized patient, the nurse, by example, can establish some guidelines for teaching the patient to weigh himself daily at home. These criteria for accurate weighing include the following:

[15] Abbey, op. cit., p. 78.
[16] Mikal, op. cit., pp. 93–98, 407–409.
[17] Guyton, op. cit., pp. 1004–1005.

1. Obtain and record weight on admission (or discharge as the case may be) as a base-line measurement.
2. Obtain and record weight at the same time daily.
3. Use the same scale daily.
4. Balance the scale before use.
5. Have patient wear approximately the same amount of clothing each day when weighed.

ASSESSMENT

Assessment by the nurse does not imply merely an evaluation of the relevance and meaning of what she observes. Assessment also means that the nurse, through her knowledge, observations, and ability to draw relationships, can anticipate the kinds of observations and actions she should make in the future. Assessment is usually carried out by relating information obtained from the patient, the patient's chart, and the nursing observations (see Figure 6–2).

Diagnosis

In the assessment of both the patient and her own observations, one of the first relationships the nurse seeks to identify is the actual or anticipated effect of the patient's diagnosis on his fluid and electrolyte balance. She asks herself, "How may the patient's clinical state affect his renal, respiratory, or circulatory function?" She asks herself, "What sequelae may accompany the apparent or suspected disease?" For example, upon admission of a patient with burns of the chest and arms, the nurse not only observes urinary output and changes in the circumference of the patient's extremities as measures of fluid loss, she also anticipates and is alert for the onset of certain additional sequelae such as respiratory distress.[18] Aside from maintaining an airway as a lifesaving measure, the nurse recognizes that any prolonged interference with the patient's ability to exchange oxygen and carbon dioxide can lead to respiratory acidosis. In the burned patient,

[18] Larson, op. cit., p. 320.

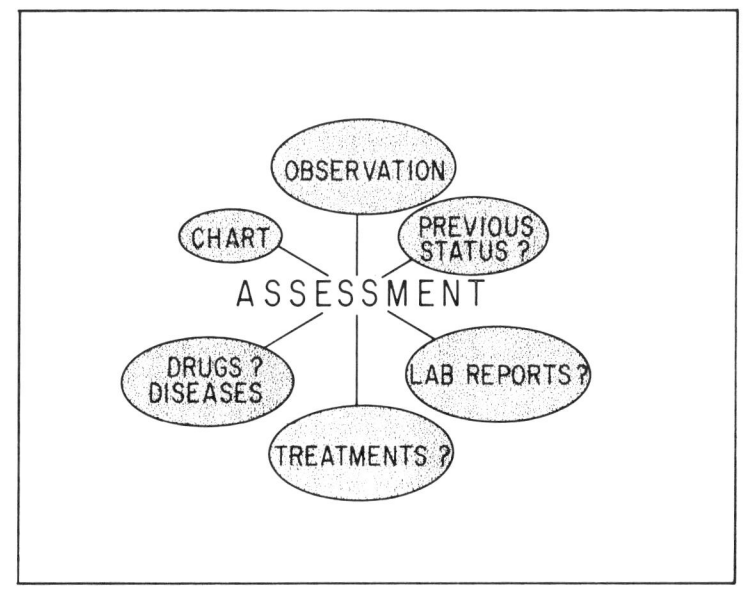

Figure 6–2 *Assessment.*

therefore, respiration distress can be particularly threatening since renal function may also be impaired, thus further affecting the patient's capacity for restoration of acid-base balance.

Previous and Present Health Status

The history of the patient's previous health status as well as of the onset of his present illness yields much information which helps the nurse in assessment of fluid and electrolyte balance. Some relevant information which may be found in these sources are these:

1. Age of the patient
2. Eating habits (history of decreased or restricted food intake)

3. Drinking habits (consumption of alcohol)
4. Medications being taken such as diuretics or laxatives
5. Use of addictive drugs
6. History of vomiting and diarrhea
7. History of recent surgery

Some of these facts may seem far removed from the nurse's assessment of the patient but indeed they are not. While the eating habits of the patient have an obvious bearing on his nutritional status, other facts such as drinking habits or use of addictive drugs may not be recognized as being relevant to fluid and electrolyte balance. The patient with cirrhosis of the liver is a potential bleeder. The patient who has been using addictive drugs has potential liver dysfunction and may also be a potential bleeder. The drug addict during withdrawal will lose large volumes of water as well as electrolytes through sweat. The alcoholic during acute withdrawal may demonstrate water retention rather than dehydration, so that close observation should be made for overhydration when such a patient is treated with intravenous fluids.[19]

Medical Treatment

An important ultimate goal for the nurse as she makes her assessment is the recognition of relationships between the patient's treatment and the actual or potential problems of fluid and electrolyte balance.

Medications such as diuretics, vasodilators, corticosteroids, potassium salts, ammonium salts, cathartics, exchange resins, antacids, digitalis and other cardiac glycosides, and central nervous system depressants may all have effects on the patient's fluid or electrolyte balance. Obviously vasopressor agents are intimately related to the patient's fluid balance. The effects of other medica-

[19] James Beard and David H. Knott, "Fluid and Electrolyte Balance During Acute Withdrawal in Chronic Alcoholic Patients," *JAMA*, 204(2): 133–139, 1968.

tions, such as central nervous system depressants on respiration, may be less obvious and in this they perhaps constitute more of a threat to the patient. In assessing the possible effects of medications and, therefore, identifying the necessary observations to be made, the nurse must again take into consideration the patient's diagnosis, and his present and past health status. In addition, a knowledge of the drug dosage, frequency, and mode of administration, as well as the time at which the last dose was received, is important in assessment of the effects of medications on fluid and electrolyte balance.

Immobilization due to organic dysfunction, bed rest, or use of casts as treatment has concomitant effects on fluid shifts and volume, and on electrolyte excretion and retention. The nurse observes the immobilized patient for changes associated with potassium excretion, sodium excretion, and those associated with venous stasis.

Preparation of patients for surgery and treatment with enemas and cathartics can lead to potassium depletion and fluid imbalance. As has been mentioned, gastrointestinal intubation, suction, and drainage can deplete the body of electrolytes and fluids. Irrigation of "-ostomies" also falls in this category of treatments which may potentiate electrolyte imbalance (see Table 4–2, p. 38).

During parenteral fluid therapy the nurse's observations become of paramount importance. Here, the observed changes in the patient's physical appearance, activity, urinary output, and vital signs are critical in assisting the doctor in evaluating the course of therapy.

Treatment of patients with concentrated solute solutions such as tube feedings should alert the nurse to observe for loss of body fluid and high blood electrolytes.

Clinical Laboratory Reports

The nurse must be able to recognize the important elements in any laboratory report and identify deviations from normal ranges. This knowledge will aid her in assessing observations and anticipating future observations.

In relation to fluid and electrolytes it is of critical importance that she familiarize herself with the following types of information:

Laboratory studies	Normal range
Blood Chemistries*	
Potassium (K+)	3.8–5.5 mEq/liter
Sodium (Na+)	136–146 mEq/liter
Chloride (Cl−)	100–106 mEq/liter
Calcium (Ca+)	4.5–5.5 mEq/liter
Carbon dioxide combining power (CO_2)	25–32 mEq/liter
Venous Blood Gases†	
Partial pressure carbon dioxide (pCO_2)	40–41 mm Hg
Partial pressure oxygen (pO_2)	35–40 mm Hg
Hydrogen ion concentration (pH)	7.36
Hemogram‡	
Hematocrit (HCT) reading	
Males	42–52 percent
Females	38–48 percent
Urinalysis¶	
Specific gravity	1.015–1.020
Hydrogen ion concentration (pH)	4.5–8.0 (usually acid, i.e., less than 7.0)
Urine sodium (Na+)	(Values obtained in 24-hour urine specimens whose results are significant only in relation to other data)
Urine potassium (K+)	

* Lillian S. Brunner et al., *Textbook of Medical-Surgical Nursing*, J. B. Lippincott Company, Philadelphia, pp. 81, 110–111.
† Carol Betson, "Blood Gases," *American Journal of Nursing*, 68(5): 1011, 1968.
‡ Brunner, op. cit., p. 111.
¶ Ibid., pp. 29, 70, 75.

Most laboratory reports include the normal ranges so that the nurse can easily identify deviations from the normal range. However, not all institutions have laboratory report sheets which include, on one sheet, reports made on several dates. In order for the nurse to assess fully the implications of any one report she needs to be aware of previous reports.

Intake and Output

The intake and output record for the patient provides both a guide for the doctor in planning fluid replacement and a means for the nurse to assess any observations she has made. The record is assessed not only in terms of those obvious gains and losses recorded, such as oral and intravenous intake of fluids, and urinary, gastrointestinal, and perspiration losses, but also in light of the patient's respiratory rate. Further, assessment of intake and output takes into consideration losses prior to hospitalization and a review of daily records from the time of the patient's hospitalization.

GROUPING OBSERVATIONS

Assessment of observations requires that one group the observations and recognize the importance of the time element.

Consider a patient with a falling blood pressure with no overt signs of bleeding: What is his diagnosis? For example, is hypotension a usual concomitant to the patient's disease entity? Has he received treatments or medications which may be accompanied by loss or retention of fluid or electrolytes? Has he received anesthetics, bowel preparation, or enemas? Has an instrument been inserted into the gastrointestinal tract? Have intravenous fluids been given? What kinds and amounts of intravenous fluid has the patient received and over what period of time? Was the patient on a "nothing-by-mouth" (NPO) order for a protracted period of time prior to surgery or admission? These kinds of questions help the nurse to rapidly but astutely assess the patient's body responses and to determine a course of action.

Another example of grouping observations might be the association of signs of dehydration or fluid loss with age, weight, history of absence or presence of preoperative vomiting or low preoperative intake, decreased postoperative urinary output, or elevated hematocrit. Again, the amount, kind, and rate of flow of intravenous fluids received are considerations. Another example might be the association of a drop in blood pressure with the presence of pain or fear, decreased urinary output, and the absence of obvious avenues of fluid loss such as gastric suction or wound exudate.

The time element must be considered, that is, when the observed symptoms actually began, what went before, and what has happen since.

Observation for fluid imbalance is particularly important in the care of the patient in the intensive care unit, coronary care unit, burn unit, hemodialysis unit, and the recovery room. For a more detailed discussion of observations in these specialized areas, a bibliography is included at the end of this book.

Once the nurse has made her assessment, she is ready to take action. Depending upon the findings of the problem-solving activity in which she has been engaged, her decision may be, in fact, to take no action.

SEVEN
THE NURSE'S ROLE IN HELPING TO MEET PATIENT AND FAMILY NEEDS

In the case of patients with real or potential fluid or electrolyte imbalance, independent nursing intervention primarily involves communication among the nurse, the patient, the patient's family, and other health team members (see Figure 7–1). Additionally, the nurse must provide for adequate oral intake of fluids when appropriate. Measures to combat the effects of immobilization should be developed jointly by the physician and nurse. However, the nurse is primarily responsible for the implementation of these measures.

Dependent nursing actions primarily involve making and reporting astute and accurate observations and assisting the doctor in the safe administration of replacement fluids and electrolytes.

MAINTAINING INTAKE AND OUTPUT

The nurse's role in maintaining intake, aside from intravenous fluid replacement, includes the provision of adequate oral intake

COMMUNICATE

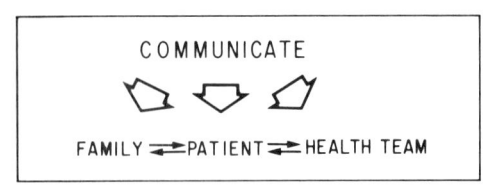

FAMILY ⇌ PATIENT ⇌ HEALTH TEAM

Figure 7-1 *Communication.*

of fluid. The decision as to what constitutes adequate intake may be within the nurse's province when the patient's doctor has made no specific recommendations. In making this determination the nurse must consider the food the patient has eaten as well as his urinary, fecal, gastrointestinal, and insensible losses, particularly visible sweat. Normally, patients drink 1500 to 2000 cc of water per day. Another 250 cc of water is ingested in food, and additional water is liberated in the oxidation of food at the rate of 10 cc of water per 100 calories of fat, carbohydrate, or protein ingested. The patient's output should be evaluated in terms of the required intake and additional fluids given as necessary. Temperature elevations in the patient or the environment, for example, usually necessitate increased intake of fluids unless contraindicated by the physician's orders. Each degree of body elevation of temperature causes vaporization of approximately 1000 cc of water from the body daily. Visible sweat over 24 hours equals a loss of 1000 to 2000 cc. Patients receiving no food continue to need water since approximately 1000 cc of water from metabolic processes may be lost in a day by urinary excretion, even under conditions of no intake.[1] Because of this, intravenous fluids are necessary for the patient receiving no fluid by mouth. Also, for the patient who has had fluids withheld in preparation for diagnostic tests, fluids must be replaced to equal concurrent losses and losses sustained during the "nothing-by-mouth" preparation period.

A variety of nursing actions may be used to promote urinary output. These may include running water within the patient's hear-

[1] Mikal, op. cit., pp. 4-5.

ing, giving the patient a drink of water when appropriate, pouring warm water over the genitalia, and helping the patient sit or walk whenever possible. Decreased urinary output should be investigated since it may indicate that the patient is experiencing urinary retention. Signs of distention of the bladder, symptoms of urinary frequency with decreased output, or symptoms of tenesmus should be drawn to the physician's attention since catheterization may be indicated.

Communication between the nurse, patient, and the patient's family involves several factors. It is important first that the patient and his family be aware of the relationship between adequate intake and output as well as the patient's diagnosis and his potential prognosis. A simple explanation that urinary output is an indication of bodily function and therefore must be observed and recorded will serve to enlist the aid of both patient and family in this respect. Again, the patient and his family must understand the need to maintain or restrict intake of fluids. A vomiting patient might receive the following explanations if they are consistent with the doctor's orders:

> Mr. Jones, when you bring up liquids from your stomach the body loses not only fluid but also important substances which are needed by the body. The doctor wants you to try to replace your losses by drinking water and juices whenever possible. We will need to know how much fluid you are losing; therefore, we must measure anything you bring up and also the amount of urine you pass. By noting the amount of urine we can tell how well the body is acting on its own to balance the fluid lost with the fluid taken in. I will leave an emesis basin here and a urinal. Please use the emesis basin if you feel sick to your stomach but pass all your urine in the urinal. I'll place your buzzer here where you can reach it easily and you can call for the nurse to remove the basin or urinal as soon as you use it. In this way you will not have these fluids sitting here at the bedside. In addition we will know how much fluid you are losing hour by hour.

The time and thought required for such an explanation goes a long way toward reassuring the patient of the nurse's concern for him and at the same time it facilitates the treatment of fluid and electrolyte imbalance should it arise.

TEACHING THE PATIENT INDEPENDENT ACTION

When a patient who may later have fluid or electrolyte imbalances is being discharged, the nurse should, where appropriate, help him and his family understand the early signs of fluid and electrolyte imbalance. Such patients include those receiving drugs such as diuretics (see Table 7–1), potassium replacements, or adrenocorticosteroids. The administration of adrenocorticosteroids may result in potassium depletion and sodium retention. The patient receiving digitalis glycosides, which are capable of inducing potassium depletion, may experience digitalis toxicity with therapeutic doses. Thus teaching the symptoms of both potassium depletion and digitalis toxicity is of prime importance for patients who have been instructed to take such drugs at home. They should also receive instruction regarding foods high in potassium and low in sodium. Such foods include dried prunes, apricots, and peaches, raisins, molasses, bananas, salt-free tomato juice, orange juice, bitter chocolate, instant coffee, grape juice, Coca-Cola, and salt-free milk.[2]

Foods high in potassium include the following:

1. Foods high in protein
2. Nonstarchy vegetables
3. Most whole fruits if fresh or dried
4. Fresh fruit juices, except apple and cranberry
5. Nuts
6. Milk solids
7. Germ of cereal grains

[2] Lilly Research Laboratories, "Clinical Application of Fluid and Electrolyte Balance," *Physicians Bulletin*, 26(1): 17, 1961.

Table 7–1 *Classification of Common Diuretics and Their Possible Complications*

Generic name	Trade name	Action	Possible complication
Thiazides		Increases excretion of sodium and chlorides	Potassium depletion
Hydrochlorothiazide	Esidrix Butiserpazide Caplaril Anhydron Cyclex Diutensin Dyazide Esimil Aldactazide (see Aldactone) Butizide Hydro-Diuril Hydropres Ser-Ap-Es		
Chlorothiazide	Diupres Diuril		
Trichlormethiazide	Metahydrin Metatensin Naquanil Naqua		
Cyclothiazide	Anhydron Anhydron K Anhydron KR		
Benzthiazide	Aquatag Exna Enduronyl Enduron Exna-R		
Bendroflumethiazide	Benuron Naturetin Rautrax		

Table 7–1 Classification of Common Diuretics and Their Possible Complications (continued)

Generic name	Trade name	Action	Possible complication
Hydroflumethiazide	Saluron		
Polythiazide	Renese		
Acetazolamide	Diamox	Inhibits carbonic anhydrase	Potassium depletion and metabolic acidosis
Triamterine	Dyrenium	Reduces potassium transport to renal tubular lumen, thus increasing sodium loss in urine	Potassium retention (Possibility of rebound potassium depletion with sudden withdrawal of drug.)
Furosemide	Lasix	Inhibits sodium and water reabsorption in proximal and distal tubules and in loop of Henle	Massive diuresis resulting in water depletion (dehydration), potassium depletion, as well as other electrolyte depletions
Sulfonamides (with diuretic action)			
Chlorthalidone	Hygroton	Inhibits carbonic anhydrase	Potassium depletion and metabolic acidosis
Quinethazone	Hydromox		Potassium depletion

Table 7–1 *Classification of Common Diuretics and Their Possible Complications (continued)*

Generic name	Trade name	Action	Possible complication
Aldactone	Aldactazide	Inhibits aldosterone's sodium retention action	In presence of a glucocorticoid may cause potassium retention
Mercurials	Mercurhydrin Meralluride Neohydrin	Depresses renal cell function, inhibiting active reabsorption of sodium in renal tubules	Sodium depletion Potassium depletion
Acid-forming salts	Ammonium	Excretion of sodium with bicarbonate	Metabolic acidosis

Source: Louis Goodman and Alfred Gilman, *The Pharmacological Basis of Therapeutics,* 3d ed., The Macmillan Company, New York, 1965; also *Physicians Desk Reference to Pharmaceutical Specialties and Biologicals,* 21st ed., Medical Economics, Oradell, N.J., 1967.

Foods low in potassium include the following:

1. Fats
2. Carbohydrates, including starchy vegetables
3. Apples and cranberries
4. Whole fruits not fresh or dried[3]

Older patients, who are predisposed to dehydration and malnutrition, as well as patients with ulcerative colitis or other diarrheic diseases, may also require explanations of symptoms of potassium and sodium depletion which they should report

[3] "Potassium Imbalance," *American Journal of Nursing,* 67(2): 358, 1967.

promptly to their physicians if and when such symptoms occur. Patients, particularly those who have a habitual dependence on laxatives, and family members who are to administer enemas also require teaching about more natural methods of controlling elimination and about the need for fluid and electrolyte (potassium) replacement when the use of laxatives and enemas cannot be avoided. Household equivalents to use in keeping intake and output records can be developed and explained to the patient and his family.

Patients who present problems in maintenance of fluid balance should be taught to observe their daily weight. The critical elements in making this observation, which were identified in the previous chapter, should be included in such a teaching plan. Emphasis should be placed upon the need to inform the physician promptly of increases or losses of weight beyond specifically defined limits established by the physician for the patient. The patient on long-term hemodialysis, for example, is said to be at an "ideal" weight when his blood pressure is normal and he is free of edema. He is expected to gain one to two kilograms, or less than one pound, between dialyses (2.2 Kg = 1 lb). Should the patient experience weight gain of one pound or more before he is scheduled to return for dialyzation, he should report to his physician.[4]

PREVENTION OF EFFECTS OF IMMOBILIZATION

The discussion here will be centered on preventing the effects of immobilization on the patient's fluid and electrolyte balance. For a more comprehensive treatment of the entire subject of immobilization and its physiological effects and the nursing implications, the reader is referred to Olsen.[5]

Immobilization has certain effects on the human body which specifically interfere with the maintenance of fluid and electrolyte

[4] Joann Albers, "Evaluation of Blood Volume in Patients on Hemodialysis," *American Journal of Nursing*, 68(8): 1679, 1969.
[5] Olsen, op. cit., pp. 780–797.

balance. The nurse must be able to explain these effects to the patient in a simple and understandable manner in order to solicit his participation in a plan to prevent their onset.

Prevention of Cardiovascular Effects

Decreased general skeletal muscle tone and loss of venopressor mechanisms which assist in venous return of blood from the lower extremities develop in the immobilized patient. There is also a redistribution of body fluid from the circulating blood volume into other parts of the body. The end result of such shifts in fluid volume is an increase in cardiac workload.[6,7,8]

The nurse can help prevent loss of muscle tone and promote muscular pressure on veins by including passive and active range of joint motion as well as isometric exercises in the plan of care. Self-care by the patient should be encouraged to the maximum permitted.[9]

Prevention of Respiratory Effects

A decrease in respiratory movement and stasis of secretions in the immobilized patient can lead to increased carbon dioxide concentrations in the blood and tissue hypoxia (decreased oxygen). In the absence of intervention, respiratory acidosis and death may be the ultimate outcome.

In addition to describing and reporting her observations, the nurse should routinely help the patient turn, cough, and breathe deeply. Teaching the patient the necessity for frequent turning,

[6] Ibid., pp. 781–782.
[7] F. B. Vogt et al., "The Effects of Bedrest on Various Parameters of Physiological Function Part XI. The Effect of Bedrest on Blood Volume, Urinary Volume, and Urinary Electrolyte Excretion," *NASA Contractor Report,* NASA CR-181, N.A.S.A., Washington, D.C., April, 1965, pp. 1–2, 19, 22.
[8] William A. Spencer, "Physiologic Concepts of Immobilization," *Archives of Physical Medicine and Rehabilitation,* 46(1A): 9–94, 1965.
[9] Olsen, op. cit., p. 782.

sitting if permitted, and stretching at regular and frequent intervals calls for the intelligent application or use of communication skills.[10] The patient should know why such activity is necessary, and he may need to be reassured that such activity will not be harmful in other ways. The patient, his family, the doctor, and the nurse should discuss this problem jointly and define the limits and advantages of such activity.

The nurse may teach the patient to use abdominal, diaphragmatic, and intercostal muscles to deepen inhalation and prolong expiration.[11]

Prevention of Metabolic Effects

Immobilization affects electrolyte balance because of three basic metabolic changes in the inactive supine person. One change is metabolic dysequilibrium in response to decreased metabolic rate. Catabolism, particularly protein catabolism, increases and results in an increase in excretion of electrolytes. Urinary excretion of electrolytes by the immobilized patient is well documented.[12] Secondly, sweating is increased because the supine position causes dilation of blood vessels and bedclothing prevents loss of heat by conduction and radiation. Sweat also carries with it the electrolytes sodium, potassium, and chloride (see Table 4-4). Thirdly, diurnal patterns (that is, variations in physiological functioning of the body during periods of night and day) occur when the individual is supine whether he is sleeping or not. During sleep the pattern of metabolic function is minimal so that supine individuals have altered nutritional and fluid requirements.

The nurse can help prevent some of these metabolic effects by helping the patient to be out of bed as ordered.[13] Some patients may need considerable encouragement and assistance to sit or walk after immobilization. They will complain of dizziness,

[10] Ibid., p. 784.
[11] Ibid., p. 789.
[12] Vogt, op. cit., pp. 6–19.
[13] Olsen, op. cit., pp. 793–794.

giddiness, or weakness. These symptoms are *real*. They are the result of orthostatic hypotension (that is, the effects of cardiovascular changes previously described).[14] Explanation of the symptoms as well as of the benefits of remaining upright will help the patient to persist in staying up as long as possible. It may be helpful for the patient to know that only persistent efforts to walk and sit will overcome orthostatic hypotension. In healthy young men who had been confined to bed for 21 days, it was shown that the ability of their cardiovascular system to respond was not regained for more than five weeks after activity was resumed.[15] This information has important implications for discharge teaching in regard to safety, falls, and so forth.

---

[14] Ibid., p. 781.
[15] Ibid., p. 781.

EIGHT
THE NURSE'S ROLE IN RELATION TO THAT OF OTHER HEALTH TEAM MEMBERS

The nurse serves as the leader of the nursing team and as such must obtain from and pass on to *all* team members pertinent information about the patient. The dietary aide, for example, has important information on patient intake. She should be aware of patients whose intake must be observed and have some identified avenue for making these observations known to the nurse. The paramedical personnel should know which patients may potentially experience fluid and electrolyte imbalance and which patients are already on intake and output. The nursing conference, the daily report, and the Kardex are used for sharing information on the patient's fluid and electrolyte balance. In addition, aids to accurate intake and output should be posted at the bedside, on the chart, and on the Kardex. A list in the utility room of patients on intake and output is also often helpful.

Common errors of intake and output include the following

(see Table 8–1): lack of a standard measurement for intake, loss of specimens, and omission of important observations on the chart. All personnel should have access to a standard of measurement, preferably in patients' rooms. All containers which may be used for distribution or collection of fluids should be marked with their volume capacity indicated in cubic centimeters or ounces or both. Frequent reminders, when necessary, should be made to all personnel of the importance of reporting and recording visible perspiration, liquid feces, vomitus, and gastric drainage, as well as fistular, wound, and other drainages as they occur. All personnel must also know which patients require increased fluids and which must have a restricted oral intake. Agreement among nursing personnel must be reached as to a method and schedule for charting intake and output, particularly of intravenous fluids.

Communication between the nurse and doctor is of para-

Table 8–1 *Intake and Output Errors and Their Causes*

Error	Cause
Inaccurate charting	Failure to record losses (perspiration, urine, liquid feces, vomitus)
	Failure to record food intake
	Failure to record daily weight
	Nonstandard methods for recording intravenous administration
Inaccurate measurement	Nonstandard containers for distribution and collection of fluids
	Poor approximation of water content of ice chips
Inaccurate fluid administration	Failure to give or restrict fluids as ordered or as necessary
	Failure to administer intravenous fluids promptly on schedule

mount importance in maintenance of the patient's fluid and electrolyte balance. The necessity for accurate recording and verbal reporting of food intake, daily weight changes, visible perspiration, and other significant changes in the patient cannot be emphasized too greatly. Verbal reporting is especially important if the doctor is not accustomed to finding such observations recorded in the nurse's notes. The nurse should obtain information from the doctor about the patient's condition which will alert her to anticipate changes in the patient. For example, she should ask for his interpretation of the significance of changes in sodium, chloride, and potassium levels and changes in arterial gas levels or CO_2 combining power.

FLUID REPLACEMENT THERAPY

The nurse in a hospital or a nursing home is also responsible for administering fluids in prescribed percentages, kinds, and amounts at safe flow rates. The doctor should be requested to write specific orders for flow rate or the period of time over which the fluid should be administered, since he has a deeper understanding of the patient's condition and of the fluids to be administered. The nurse, however, is legally responsible for her actions when administering intravenous fluids. Therefore, a discussion of her role in respect to intravenous fluid administration is in order.

Recognition of the tonicity of prescribed fluids provides some guidelines for their administration. Isotonic solutions generally may be administered more rapidly than hypotonic or hypertonic solutions. Isotonic saline may be administered at a rate of 600 cc per hour; however, during emergencies such as traumatic shock or hemorrhagic shock up to 2000 cc may be administered in one hour to support circulating blood volume. In the absence of renal impairment or other contraindications, isotonic solutions containing glucose may be run at a maximum rate of 0.5 gm of glucose per kilogram body weight per hour. In a 165-lb man the calculated rate is as follows:

0.5 gm glucose/kg body weight/hour (2.2 kg = 1 lb)

$$0.5 \text{ gm glucose}/2.2 \overline{\smash{\big)}165.0}^{\,75.0 \text{ kg}} \text{ lb/hr}$$

0.5 gm glucose/75 kg/hr = 37.5 gm glucose in 1 hr

One thousand cc of 5 percent glucose in water contains 5 gm of glucose in each 100 cc of solution. In order for the patient to obtain 37.5 gm of glucose in one hour, 750 cc of 5 percent glucose and water may be given to a 165-lb man in 1 hour if no renal or cardiac complications exist.

$$5 \text{ gm} \overline{\smash{\big)}37.5 \text{ gm}}^{\,7.5 \times 100 \text{ cc} = 750.0 \text{ cc}}$$
$$\underline{35}$$
$$25$$
$$\underline{25}$$

More rapid administration of glucose is inadvisable since circulatory glucose then would exceed the renal threshold for sugar and the extra sugar would be excreted with large amounts of urine. Both fluid and serum potassium levels also can be seriously lowered in this manner.

Hypertonic solutions such as 10 percent fructose in water or 5 percent glucose in lactated Ringer's solution should be given at a rate of about 200 cc per hour. More rapid administration may cause a sudden shift of intracellular water into the extracellular spaces. Such a shift would subsequently increase the blood volume. The patient's heart, if unable to accommodate the sudden extra workload, may fail, resulting in pulmonary edema and death. Since hypertonic replacement solutions may be relatively hypotonic to intracellular fluid in dehydrated patients, these solutions may be infused at slightly faster rates in such patients.

Hypotonic solutions such as 0.45 percent saline in water or 2.5 percent dextrose in water also must be given at slower rates than isotonic solutions; however, they may be administered more rapidly than hypertonic solutions. The safe rate of 250 to 400 cc per hour prevents a sudden shift of extracellular water into the cells, thus preventing a precipitate drop in blood volume which could cause cardiac failure, shock, and death. Another result of a rapid or slow shift of fluids intracellularly is the development of water intoxication; death may follow.

When adjusting flow rates, the nurse should be aware that because of the variation in the size of the outlet, different intravenous administration sets will vary in the numbers of drops which equal 1 cc. For example, the Abbott Venopak is calibrated to provide 15 gtt = 1 cc, whereas in the Abbott blood administration set approximately 10 gtt = 1 cc. Baxter sets deliver 10 gtt = 1 cc. Pediatric sets range from 50 gtt = 1 cc to 60 gtt = 1 cc.

A chart can be developed based on the drop rate of the administration set so as to compute desired drops per minute necessary to infuse specific amounts of fluid over varying time periods. For example, the doctor may order 2000 cc of fluid to be given over a 16-hour period. If the nurse knows that the administration set delivers 10 gtt = 1 cc, she may calculate the flow rate using this formula:

$$\begin{aligned}\text{gtt/min over 16 hr to equal 2000 cc} &= \frac{\text{Total volume to be infused} \times \text{gtt/cc}}{\text{Total time of infusion in min}} \\ &= \frac{2000 \times 10}{960} \\ &= 20.7 \text{ or } 21 \text{ gtt/min for 16 hr}\end{aligned}$$

The nurse can prepare charts which identify differing flow rates and place the charts near the intravenous stock cabinets for ready reference.

Some general statements of fact and precautions in regard to fluid replacement therapy are as follows:

1. Usually, infusion must be done at a slow rate in aged and very young patients.
2. Urinary output must be observed along with flow rate. The rate must be reduced and the physician consulted in these circumstances:
   a. Urinary output drops below 50 cc per hour.
   b. Urinary output exceeds infused fluid in any given period (e.g., per hour).
3. Patients with renal or cardiac dysfunction should be closely observed for signs of onset of overhydration when receiving parenteral fluids.
4. Intravenous administration of potassium is governed by the following precautions:
   a. Adequate urinary output must be established and maintained.
   b. No more than 30 mEq of potassium chloride (KCl) should be infused in 1 hour.
   c. A potassium concentration of no more than 40 mEq per liter should be maintained.
   d. No more than 80 mEq of KCl should be given in any one infusion (that is, a maximum of 2 liters of intravenous fluid with KCl administered consecutively).
   e. Never infuse a concentrated solution of potassium directly into the vein.
   f. Note laboratory results and draw the doctor's attention immediately to abnormalities in serum potassium levels.[1]
5. Often mechanical factors will interfere with the maintenance of the desired flow rate. Such factors include these:
   a. Movement of the needle so that the lumen is obstructed by the venous wall.
   b. A change in the height of the infusion bottle or the patient's bed. The greater the distance between the patient and the bottle the faster the rate of flow.

[1] Abbey, op. cit., p. 83.

c. The lumen of the needle may be obstructed by a small clot of blood.

The hazards of replacement therapy, aside from those already noted such as water intoxication and potassium intoxication, include air embolism and pulmonary edema.

Cyanosis, hypotension, weak rapid pulse, and loss of consciousness in a patient receiving infusions are symptoms of air embolism. The greatest possibilities for this exist when a Y-type of infusion set is used for the administration of blood which is to be followed by saline (see Figure 8–1). When the patient has received

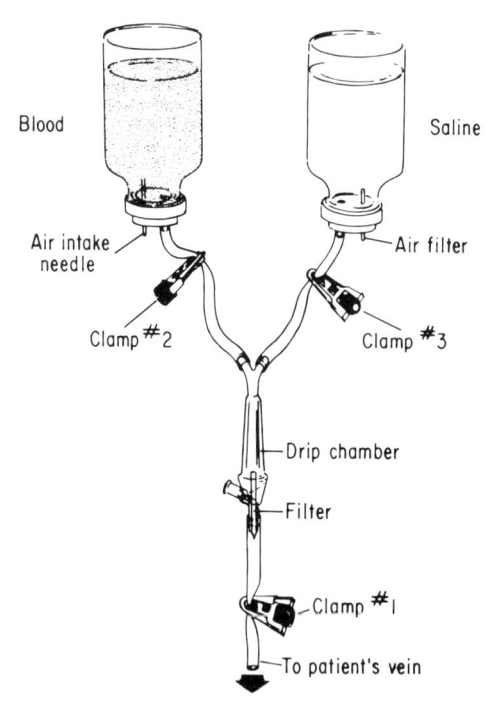

Figure 8–1 *Close #2 clamp before opening #3 clamp to prevent air embolism.*

the entire amount of blood, the tubing leading from that bottle should be clamped off completely before the stopcock controlling the saline is opened; otherwise air may enter the patient's vein from the empty blood bottle. A second important precaution is that the extremity receiving blood should not be raised above the level of the heart, since to do so causes negative venous pressure and results in air entering the venous system if there are defects in the infusion apparatus.

Shortness of breath with increased respiratory rate, increased blood pressure, and venous distention are signs of circulatory overload—the forerunner of pulmonary edema. Should such symptoms occur during the administration of intravenous fluids, the infusion should be stopped and the physician notified immediately.

PART THREE
APPROACH TO CLINICAL STUDY
FOR THE STUDENT AND THE TEACHER

NINE
A PROBLEM-SOLVING APPROACH TO NURSING ASSESSMENT

In each of the following situations, the student will have an opportunity to use knowledge gained from the text in order to identify the appropriate nurse action. Related questions are designed to encourage the student to use other reference sources, thus widening the command of resources in background information.

SITUATION A

Will Brown, age 18, was in an automobile accident. He was brought into the emergency room in a state of shock. The doctor ordered 1000 cc normal saline to be administered intravenously at once. Later, internal hemorrhage was suspected, and blood was administered to the patient.

Discuss each of the following important points:

1. What are the symptoms of shock? What causes these symptoms?
2. What is a safe rate of flow for the administration of normal saline under the foregoing circumstances?
3. What is the tonicity of normal saline? How does this influence the rate at which it may be administered?
4. What are the other factors which influence the rate of administration of saline? What factors may affect the safe administration of the blood? What danger exists when blood administration is completed and saline infusion is started?
5. What other clinical states may result in shock-like symptoms?

SITUATION B

Mr. Wilson, age 82, was admitted to the hospital with a history of increasing respiratory difficulty including gurgling rales and dyspnea unrelated to exertion. Mr. Wilson appeared slightly dazed and lethargic. He had a cough productive of thick sputum. He was diagnosed as having respiratory acidosis secondary to pulmonary emphysema.

1. What kinds of blood tests may be ordered to follow the course of the patient's illness? Why would a CO_2 combining power test show a drop below normal, whereas arterial gas studies of carbon dioxide might demonstrate a rise above normal or a drop below normal?
2. What is the relationship of the pathological changes in the respiratory system of the emphysematous patient and the development of respiratory acidosis?
3. Should intravenous fluids be ordered for this patient? What danger of complication is inherent?
4. How does this patient's age affect the possibility of complications accompanying intravenous fluid administration?
5. What nursing observations are of paramount importance during the administration of intravenous fluid to this patient? Why?

SITUATION C

Mrs. Long, age 35, was admitted to the hospital with a diagnosis of chronic renal insufficiency and malignant hypertension. The student nurse was assigned to assist the patient with morning care.

1. What symptoms related to electrolyte imbalance might the student expect to see because of Mrs. Long's kidney disease?
2. What observations regarding urinary output would be pertinent? Why?
3. The patient is nauseated and vomits. How might this affect her electrolyte balance?
4. What specific precautions and observations are necessary when this patient receives intravenous fluids?
5. What factors are considered in adjustment of intravenous flow rates for this patient?

SITUATION D

Miss Conlon, age 28, is admitted with a history of intermittent diarrhea over the preceding 6 months following the death of her mother. The patient's weight on admission was 86 pounds. She is diagnosed as having ulcerative colitis. Intravenous fluids are ordered immediately and include 1000 cc of 2.5 percent dextrose in 0.45 saline, and 1000 cc of 5 percent dextrose in water with 40 mEq per liter of potassium added, to be administered over 12 hours.

1. What is the danger implicit in rapid administration of the 2.5 percent dextrose in 0.45 saline? Why?
2. What instructions should the nurse give to the nursing team in relation to Miss Conlon's intake and output? In relation to her weight?
3. Which electrolytes are lost in the greatest amounts in diarrheal stools?

4. Why does the nurse expect this patient to have decreased urinary output?

5. Why does the nurse expect that the urinary output will not fall below 600 cc per 24 hours, even if the patient is receiving no fluids?

6. What is the flow rate per minute necessary to carry out the doctor's orders if the administration set delivers 10 gtt = 1 cc?

7. Should dehydration of this patient continue unresponsive to treatment, what symptoms may the patient demonstrate? Why?

8. Prednisone therapy is prescribed on the patient's discharge. What patient teaching relative to fluid and electrolyte balance is necessary regarding this drug? Why is this teaching especially significant for this patient?

SITUATION E

Mr. Jones, age 45, was admitted to the hospital with a history of dyspnea and syncope. On a previous admission he had been treated for a myocardial infarction. His temperature was normal. His pulse was arrhythmic and slow. At home he had been taking a digitalis preparation daily and received a mecurial diuretic three times a week from the public health nurse. He was diagnosed as having decompensating congestive heart failure and possible digitalis toxicity.

1. What is the relationship of digitalis toxicity to mecurial diuretics? What other drugs bear the same relationship? Why?

2. What major points would you include in a teaching plan for patients and their families when the patient is given prescriptions for digitalis and diuretic preparations on discharge?

3. What are the early signs of potassium depletion?

4. How can you find out which foods Mr. Jones can eat which are low in salt and high in potassium?

5. During the intravenous replacement of potassium for any patient, what are the precautions of which the nurse should be aware?

6. Name some commonly available mecurial diuretic preparations. Are some diuretic preparations (mecurial or otherwise) less likely than others to cause potassium depletion? What, if any, are these preparations?

SITUATION F

Marion Wilson, age 35, was admitted with severe burns of the anterior trunk and arms (approximately 27 percent of the body surface). The doctor's orders included the following: "Insert large-bore polyethylene catheter into the saphenous vein. Give 600 cc plasma for falling B/P with decreased urinary output, otherwise run in lactated Ringer's solution 1000 cc. Regulate intravenous flow to maintain urine output 25 to 50 cc/hr Stat. Weigh patient Stat. Insert Foley catheter. Elevate arms. NPO except for ice chips. Nasogastric tube for vomiting or abdominal distention."

1. Why is it necessary to give this patient plasma or other colloid infusions?

2. What is the relationship of the falling blood pressure and decreased urinary output to the need for colloid infusions?

3. What is the importance of weighing the patient as early as possible on admission?

4. Why might this patient vomit or have abdominal distention? Why is she on "NPO" orders? How can you measure the amount of water taken in as ice chips?

5. What solution should be used to irrigate the nasogastric tube if it is inserted? Why?

6. Urinary output above 50 cc per hour is significant and calls for nurse action. In this instance what is the significance and what should you do? Does the patient's age have any significance? Why?

7. Why does this patient receive lactated Ringer's solution?

8. Why is metabolic acidosis apt to develop?

9. What is the most critical nursing role in the care of this patient during the immediate period following admission?

10. What does the nurse communicate to her team to insure that the critical elements of nursing care are maintained for this patient?

SITUATION G

Mrs. Lawson, age 62, was admitted to the hospital with acute intestinal obstruction. A cecostomy was performed. Prior to admission the patient had been unable to eat for 2 days and had had a history of nausea and vomiting. Postoperatively intermittent nasogastric suction was employed.

1. What electrolytes may be lost in the cecostomy drainage?

2. What other avenues of loss of fluid and electrolytes must be considered in observing intake and output in this patient?

3. What blood chemistry reports should be observed and reported to the doctor in the event of abnormal fluctuations?

4. For what reason should irrigation of the nasogastric tube be carried out with isotonic solutions?

5. How might hypotonic solutions be introduced into this patient's gastrointestinal tract?

6. How would the introduction of hypotonic solutions into the gastrointestinal tract affect the patient?

TEN
SUGGESTIONS FOR CLINICAL TEACHING

So often the appropriate use of the clinical setting for teaching the nursing role in relation to fluid and electrolytes is misunderstood and therefore is not as effective as it might be. Faculty have a tendency to focus the student's attention on carrying out nursing functions or comprehending the patient's disease entity rather than on the more inclusive role of the nurse which will be discussed below. Fragmentation of the student's learning experience does not lend itself to imparting optimal benefits from clinical learning experiences. However, because it is difficult to avoid such fragmentation when one desires to provide experiences appropriate to the student's current level of understanding, the following suggestions are offered.

The nurse's role in relation to maintenance of the patient's fluid and electrolyte balance includes observation and assessment, identifying the patient's specific problems or needs in this area, understanding the rationale for these needs or problems, identifying appropriate nurse actions, implementing and evaluating the effects of the action on the patient's problems or needs. The evaluation process in turn leads to a renewed cycle of observation and assessment. Students are not capable of entirely fulfilling the nurse's role in their early contacts with patients for a variety of reasons. These reasons include insufficient knowledge of the usual causes and effects of electrolyte imbalance, fragmented ability to associate knowledge of fluid and electrolyte balance and imbalance with the patient's needs or problems, and insufficient skill in problem solving and ability to effectively plan the nurse actions. The student progresses from ability to observe, to ability to draw relationships, to ability to identify a course of action, and finally to ability to carry out those actions. Evaluation of the effectiveness of nurse actions in terms of changes in the patient is the most advanced step in fulfillment of the nurse's role and usually occurs late in the student's development.

Rather than treat the question of how to introduce and develop this subject matter throughout an entire program, we will deal with a general approach which may be adapted for various nursing education programs at different times, depending upon the students' levels of understanding at any particular point in the program.

When the student has completed adjunct courses or study in physiology which deals with the normal mechanisms for maintaining homeostasis, the stress response of the body, circulation, and elimination, she may then begin the study of the threats posed by certain clinical states to fluid and electrolyte balance. The student needs factual information so that she can observe and assess the patient's fluid and electrolyte balance and understand her own role in administration of fluid therapy. This content is treated extensively in a variety of nursing arts texts. Students beginning study in the care of patients with fluid and electrolyte imbalance should not be expected to fully understand the relationships between the effects of the patient's disease entity or medical therapy and his needs in maintenance of fluid and electrolyte balance. The faculty member, as she discusses the patient with the student, should identify (with the student's help if possible) the patient's needs and explain the rationale. The patients who are chosen should give clear evidence of the particular observations upon which the teacher is focusing for the student's learning experience. The student should be assisted in the assessment of her observations and then given the problem of deciding what should be done about these observations. She should also be given the problem of identifying the kinds of nursing approaches she may carry out. Subsequently, after she has had the opportunity to carry out her approaches, the student should evaluate her nursing care. This final step is reached through discussion with the instructor, who may also strengthen the evaluation with questions and comments during one-to-one or group postclinical conferences.

Study of the nurse's role in the maintenance of fluid and electrolyte balance may be introduced on any hospital unit and with any age group of patients. The instructor may select a patient who will be on the unit for at least two or three consecutive days during the period when the student is assigned to the unit for clinical experience. If it is not possible for the student to care for the same patient, patients having similar clinical pictures (not necessarily the same diagnoses) should be assigned to the student. Suitable patients for a student beginning the study of fluid and electrolyte balance include dehydrated or malnourished elderly or infant patients. Other patients presenting fluid and electrolyte problems may include those in the first or second day following uncomplicated gastrointestinal or gynecological surgery, elderly persons or infants with fever, individuals with potassium deficiencies associated with heart disease, or, finally, those with pernicious vomiting due to pregnancy or other causes. The instructor should plan to assist the student to first observe, then to assess, and later to identify and carry out other nursing actions based on her observation and assessment.

Each experience may be focused for the student by means of a teaching aid which this author terms a Focus Sheet. The student should not be responsible for fulfilling the nurse's role beyond the focus for the day unless she is further directed in her actions by the instructor. The Focus Sheet serves as a study guide and checklist before and after the clinical experience.

Having been assisted in reaching a general understanding of the relationships between the patient's present health status and a potential or actual fluid or electrolyte imbalance, the student may be given a Focus Sheet (see Focus I). She may then provide physical care for her assigned patient

Focus I *Nurse's Role in Observation of the Patient with Potential*

Objectives

To increase ability in observation and identification of the adaptive responses of individuals to changes in fluid and/or electrolyte balance by:

a. Recognizing significant changes in the physical appearance, and color, temperature, moisture of skin.
b. Recognizing significant changes in the patient's sensory status.
c. Recognizing significant changes in the patient's gastrointestinal and/or urinary output, that is, amount, frequency, consistency, odor, and color.
d. Recognizing significant changes in the color and/or texture of the mucous membranes and/or nail beds.
e. Recognizing significant changes and vital signs.

during which time she will have ample opportunity to make her observations. If her patient is receiving intravenous fluids, or has nasogastric intubation, or is on a controlled program of intake and output, the beginning student will need specific assistance and direction for giving care. Focus should be constantly directed at the student's observations rather than the functional nursing problems of caring for an intubated patient. Postconference should be given over to comparison by students of similar or differing observations and to discussion of the possible significance of their observations. At this point students may be encouraged to learn more about the patient's disease and treatment. A well-placed comment, such as, "I wonder what relationships there may be between this patient's lowered blood pressure and decreased urinary output?" or, "Could this patient's

or Actual Problems of Fluid and Electrolyte Balance

Ask yourself

a. How does the patient's skin look, feel?

b. Is the patient confused, lethargic, apathetic, apprehensive, restless?
c. Is there a decrease or increase in amount, in frequency? Is there a change in odor, in color?

d. Are membranes dry or moist, pale, blue or pink? Are nail beds pale, blue, or pink?
e. Is the blood pressure lowered? Is the pulse rapid, slow, irregular? Are the respirations rapid, deep, slow, shallow? Is the temperature elevated; if so, to what degree?

Focus II *Nurse's Role in Assessment of the Patient with Potential*

Objectives

To increase ability to assess nursing observations and to determine what should be done about them through:

a. Recognizing the relationship between the patient's diagnosis and observed changes in the patient.

b. Recognizing the relationship between patient's health history and his present illness; the relationship of his age and nutritional status to observed changes.

c. Recognizing the relationship between treatments the patient received and observed changes in the patient.

d. Recognition of the significance of laboratory reports of K^+, Na^+, Cl^- and CO_2 levels in the patient's blood and observed changes in the patient.

e. Deciding how to group observations into a meaningful picture.

f. Deciding who and when to tell about the observations.

g. Deciding what to record.

or Actual Problems of Fluid and Electrolyte Balance

Ask yourself

a. How does the patient's disease affect kidney function, physical appearance of skin, temperature, pulse, respiration? How did the patient demonstrate changes in kidney function? Was urinary output changed? Which of the observations are related to circulatory dysfunction? To skin changes?

b. Was the patient vomiting? Diaphoretic? Having diarrhea? Without food? Taking frequent enemas or laxatives? Taking diuretics before admission? Since admission? Is your patient old, young, fat, thin? On fluids or full diet?

c. What medications and/or treatments is the patient receiving? How can they affect physical appearance, sensory status, gastrointestinal and/or urinary output, vital signs? When was patient's last treatment? His last dose?

d. How do the patient's laboratory reports differ from normal? What observations should accompany these changes? Did I see them? Which of these observations might result from alterations in electrolytes? Which ones should I check on the chart? Did I compare lab reports from different dates for changes in blood levels?

e. How long have changes observed in the patient been present? When did they start? How often do they occur? Do these changes seem to relate to other information obtained about the patient?

f. To whom should I report my findings? When? Now? After care? When further observations are made?

g. What needs to go in the nurse's notes? Are these observations recorded elsewhere? Is the nurse legally responsible to put these observations on the chart? Will knowledge of these observations be helpful on Kardex, in the utility room?

Focus III *Nurse's Role in Identifying and Implementing Nurse Balance in Patients*

Objectives

1. To increase ability in identifying and interpreting patient and family needs by:

   a. Recognizing the modes, amounts, and probable electrolytic constituents of fluids taken in and eliminated by the patient.

   b. Identifying adequate oral intake of fluids when appropriate.

   c. Recognizing with accuracy factors related to the administration of parenteral fluids in the prescribed amounts at the prescribed rates when appropriate.

   d. Recognizing the patient's as well as the family's need to know early signs of fluid loss and a simple method of measuring intake and output when they are intimately involved with the patient's health supervision.

2. To increase development of communication techniques in meeting patient and family needs by:

   a. Maintaining verbal and written communication on the intake and output of the patient with appropriate members of the health team.

   b. Teaching the family, and the patient when appropriate, simple methods of measuring and recording intake and, in some instances, urinary output.

3. To increase skill in the application of basic nursing skills by:

   a. Maintaining medical asepsis in the care of drainage tubings of any type and surgical asepsis in the care of parenteral fluids and equipment before and during their use in administration.

Actions Which Assist in the Maintenance of Fluid and Electrolyte

Ask yourself

a. Did you check intake and output records, ask the family, the patient, or other personnel? What and how much has the patient eaten? Is this important?
b. What fluids were offered the patient orally? Do certain oral fluids provide more of certain electrolytes than others? Can the patient have any fluids?
c. Were intravenous fluids ordered; are they being infused? Was the infusing fluid the percent ordered? Was the rate as prescribed or within safe limits? What was the flow rate?
d. How and when would you use this information in communicating with the patient or his family? Did you plan to involve the patient and/or his explanations? Why? Why not? How can you explain the patient's need for intake and output? Intravenous fluids?

a. Did you chart the patient's intake and output? Where? To whom did you report your observations?

b. Did you actually involve the patient and/or his family? Why? Why not?

a. When were the drainage tubes and collecting equipment last changed? Were their tips contaminated during care? Did you keep irrigating equipment and solutions clean or sterile? Did you maintain sterility of tubing and bottles when changing bottles?

Focus III *Nurse's Role in Identifying and Implementing Nurse Balance in Patients (continued)*

Objectives
b. Maintaining correct flow rate.
c. Providing physical comfort for the patient, as appropriate, by helping him maintain a skin temperature and moisture as normal as possible. d. Positioning the patient for comfort as well as the maintenance of the flow of parenteral fluids and patency and/or flow of drainage tubes as necessary.

medications have affected her blood pressure or caused arrhythmic pulse rates?" often stimulates the student to seek further information or to use the information she already has in reaching a rational explanation or answer.

During the second session (not necessarily the second day—this may be a later experience) the average student usually comes to the experience with more knowledge about the patient's illness and treatments and about fluid and electrolyte imbalance. Her focus should then be directed at the assessment of her observations (see Focus II). She should be allowed ample time to observe the patient, to use the chart, and to talk with the doctor and head nurse, in order to assess her observations. *The student should be freed from the necessity of giving physical care to the patient* during this experience *if it prevents* her having time to *focus on the objective of the day*. The teacher should review the student's charting of observations for their relevance and accuracy. Close attention is given to the student's reporting. Postconference then centers on the day's experiences, the kinds of needs the patient may have in view of the student's assess-

Actions Which Assist in the Maintenance of Fluid and Electrolyte

---

Ask yourself

b. Were you able to adjust the flow rate? How was flow rate affected by patient's position? Movement? Application of the intravenous administration set? Height of bottle? Height of bed?

c. If patient's skin was cold and/or wet, what did you do? Hot and/or dry what did you do?

d. When patient was positioned, was the drainage or intravenous tubing patent? Could fluid drain through intravenous tubing or drainage tubing by gravity?

---

ment, as well as tentative nursing actions. The nursing care plan provides the student with an additional opportunity to assess her observations and to identify patient needs as well as nurse actions. It may be necessary for the instructor to provide the student with a new patient, but one with a similar clinical state, for the third focus. The third focus, again, may be dealt with in another two or three day experience. The final focus at this level is geared to helping the student carry out identified needed nurse actions (see Focus III). The student's evaluation of the effectiveness of her actions should be made during a postassignment group conference.

The instructor's evaluation of the student's performance should take place *after* completion of all learning experiences. In other words, after these three clinical focuses, the student should be given further opportunity to care for a similar patient and to then be evaluated on the progress she has made in observing, assessing observations, recognizing patient needs, and planning and carrying out nursing actions.

Fluid and electrolyte balance is of vital importance in the maintenance of life; moreover, there exists a wide variety of circumstances during which imbalance may be precipitated. Thus the nurse's understanding and application of knowledge in regard to the maintenance of fluid and electrolyte balance in patients should have a central position in all nursing practice and every nursing curriculum. It is hoped this book has served to help the nursing practitioner, student, and educator in fulfilling their goals in these respects.

BIBLIOGRAPHY

Abbey, June: "Nursing Observations of Fluid Imbalance," *Nursing Clinics of North America,* 3:1, March, 1968, pp. 77–86.

Abbott Laboratories: *Fluid and Electrolytes,* Abbott Laboratories, North Chicago, 1963.

Albers, Joann: "Evaluation of Blood Volume in Patients on Hemodialysis," *American Journal of Nursing,* 68:8, August, 1968, pp. 1677–1679.

Anderson, J. Persons et al.: "A Medical Metering Pump," *Lancet,* 1, March 25, 1961, pp. 646–647.

Baxter Laboratories: *The Fundamentals of Body Water and Electrolytes,* Baxter Laboratories, Morton Grove, Illinois, 1967.

Beard, James and David H. Knott: "Fluid and Electrolyte Balance During Acute Withdrawal in Chronic Alcoholic Patients," *Journal American Medical Association,* 204:2, April 8, 1968, pp. 133–137.

Beland, Irene L.: *Clinical Nursing,* The Macmillan Company, New York, 1965, pp. 482–557.

Best, Charles and Norman Taylor: *The Physiological Basis of Medical Practice*, 7th ed., The Williams & Wilkins Co., Baltimore, 1961.
Betson, Carol: "Blood Gases," *American Journal of Nursing*, 68:5, May, 1968, pp. 1010–1012.
Black, D. A. K.: *Essentials of Fluid Balance*, 4th ed., Blackwell Scientific Publications, Ltd., Oxford, 1967.
Bland, John H.: *Clinical Metabolism of Body Water and Electrolytes*, W. B. Saunders Company, Philadelphia, 1963, Chaps. 2, 3, 4, 6, 7, 8.
Bonsnes, R. W.: "Postoperative and Parenteral Nutrition," *Surgical Clinics of North America*, XXXVII, April, 1957, pp. 307–320.
Brunner, Lillian S., Charles Emerson, L. Kraeer Fergusen, and Doris S. Suddareth: *Textbook of Medical-Surgical Nursing*, J. B. Lippincott Company, Philadelphia, 1964, pp. 65–114, 159–185.
Dunning, M. F. and F. Pleem: "Potassium Depletion by Enemas," *American Journal of Medicine*, XX, May, 1956, pp. 789–792.
Farr, Hallon W.: "Fluid and Electrolyte Balance with Special Reference to the Gastrointestinal Tract," *American Journal of Nursing*, 59, July, 1959, pp. 827–831.
Goodman, Louis J. and Alfred Gilman: *The Pharmacological Basis of Therapeutics*, 3d ed., The Macmillan Co., New York, 1965, pp. 820–899.
Guyton, Arthur: *A Textbook of Medical Physiology*, 2d ed., W. B. Saunders Company, Philadelphia, 1961.
———: *A Textbook of Medical Physiology*, 3d ed., W. B. Saunders Company, Philadelphia, 1966, pp. 1045–1046.
Howard, John M.: "Fluid Replacement in Shock and Hemorrhage," *Journal American Medical Association*, CLXXIII, June 4, 1960, pp. 516–518.
Larson, Duane and Rita Gaston: "Current Trends in the Care of Burned Patients," *American Journal of Nursing*, 67:2, February, 1967, pp. 319–327.
Lilly Research Laboratories: "Clinical Application of Fluid and Electrolyte Balance," *Physicians Bulletin*, XXVI: 1, February, 1961.
Medical Economics: *Physician's Desk Reference to Pharmaceutical Specialties and Biologicals*, 21st ed., Medical Economics, Oradell, New Jersey, 1967.

Metheny, Norma and William Snively: *Nurses' Handbook of Fluid Balance,* J. B. Lippincott Company, Philadelphia, 1967.

Mikal, Stanley: *Homeostasis in Man,* Little, Brown and Company, Boston, 1967.

Nett, Louise and Thomas L. Petty: "Acute Respiratory Failure," *American Journal of Nursing,* 67:9, September, 1967, pp. 1847–1851.

Netter, Frank: *The Ciba Collection of Medical Diseases,* Vol. IV. *Endocrine System and Selected Metabolic Diseases,* Ciba Pharmaceutical Co., Summit, New Jersey, 1965, pp. 9, 32, 34.

Olsen, Edith, et al.: "The Hazards of Immobility," *American Journal of Nursing,* 67:4, April, 1967, pp. 781–797.

Parker, Victor et al.: "Body Water Compartments Throughout the Life Span," *Ciba Foundation Colloquia on Aging,* Vol. 4, ed. C. E. Wolenstenholme, Little, Brown and Company, Boston, 1958, pp. 102–113.

Pfizer, Spectrum: *Intravenous Technique,* Reprint, Pfizer Laboratories' Spectrum, 235 East 42d St., New York, N.Y. 10017.

"Potassium Imbalance," *American Journal of Nursing,* 67:2, February, 1967, p. 358.

Pullen, H. et al.: "Intensive I.V. Potassium Replacement Therapy," *Lancet,* 2, October 14, 1967, pp. 809–811.

Simeone, F. A.: "Shock: Its Nature and Treatment," *American Journal of Nursing,* 66:6, June, 1966, pp. 1286–1294.

Smith, Dorothy and Claudia Gips: *Care of the Adult Patient,* 2d ed., J. B. Lippincott Company, Philadelphia, 1954, pp. 122–129.

Spencer, William A., Carlos Valbona, and R. Edward Carter, Jr.: "Physiologic Concepts of Immobilization," *Archives of Physical Medicine and Rehabilitation,* 46:1-A, January, 1965, pp. 89–100.

Statland, Harry: *Fluids and Electrolytes in Practice,* 2d ed., J. B. Lippincott Company, Philadelphia, 1957.

Talbot, N. B. and R. Richie: "The Effect of Age on the Body's Tolerance for Fasting, Thirsting and Overloading with Water and Certain Electrolytes," G. E. Wolenstenholm (ed.), *Ciba Foundation Colloquia on Aging,* vol. 4, Little, Brown and Company, Boston, 1958, pp. 139–150.

Valbona, C., F. B. Vogt, D. Cardus, W. A. Spencer, and M. Walters: "The Effect of Bedrest on Various Parameters of Physiological

Function. Part I. Review of Literature on the Physiological Effects of Immobilization," *NASA Contractor Report*, NASA CR-171, National Aeronautics and Space Administration, Washington, D.C., March, 1965.

Vogt, F. B., W. A. Spencer, D. Cardus, and C. Valbona: "The Effects of Bedrest on Various Parameters of Physiological Function. Part XI. The Effect of Bedrest on Blood Volume, Urinary Volume, and Urinary Electrolyte Excretion," *NASA Contractor Report*, NASA CR-181, National Aeronautics and Space Administration, Washington, D.C., April, 1965.

———: "The Effects of Bedrest on Various Parameters of Physiological Function. Part VI. The Effect of the Performance of Periodic Flack Maneuvers on Preventing Cardiovascular Deconditioning of Bedrest," *NASA Contractor Report*, NASA CR-176, National Aeronautics and Space Administration, Washington, D.C., July, 1965.

INDEX

Acid-base balance:
  bicarbonate ions, 37
  buffers, 30–32
  hydrogen ions, 30, 37
  pH, 30
    normal range, arterial blood, 30
  regulation of, 30–33
    renal, 24–27, 37, 39
    respiratory, 32, 37, 59–60
  relationship to cell function, 30
Acidosis:
  defined, 30–31
  metabolic, 51–52

Acidosis:
  respiratory, 51, 59–60
Active transport:
  defined, 12–13
  in renal tubules, 12
ADH (see Antidiuretic hormone)
Alcoholism, water retention in, 66
Aldosterone:
  adrenal cortex, 28
  function, 28, 29
  rate of secretion, 28–29
  relationship to potassium, 28
  relationship to sodium, 28

Alkalosis:
 defined, 30
 metabolic, 51–52
 respiratory, 52, 59, 60
Anions, 20
Antidiuretic hormone (ADH):
 function of, 26–28
 relationship to urinary output, 27–28
 release, 26
 secretion, 27
 source, 26–27
 storage, 26
Assessment of patients:
 problem-solving in: with acute intestinal obstruction, 98
  with burns, 97–98
  with chronic renal insufficiency, 95
  with congestive heart failure, 96–97
  with digitalis toxicity, 96–97
  with respiratory acidosis, 93–94
  with shock, 93
  with ulcerative colitis, 95–96
 role of nurse in, 64–70
  defined, 64
  relationship of: diagnosis, medical, 64–65
   health status, 65–66
   intake and output, 69
   laboratory tests, 67–68

Assessment of patients:
 role of nurse in: relationship of: treatment, medical, 66–67

Bicarbonate ions, 37
Blood chemistries, 68
Blood pressure, 60–61
Body fluid:
 age, 7
 blood pressure changes, 38
 circulation, 24
 decreases, 39–40, 45–47
 increases, 41, 44–45
 loss of, 34–35, 39–40
 movement of, 10–20
 obligatory loss of, 34–35
 observations related to, 56–63
 osmolarity, 15
 temperature in, 59
 tissues, influence of, 7
 toxicity of, 15–18
Buffers, 30–32

Calcium, normal blood concentrations, 68
Calcium imbalance, symptoms of, 50
Carbon dioxide:
 normal blood concentrations, 68
  combining power, 68
  partial pressure, 68
  venous gases, 68

INDEX

Carbonic acid, 31–32
Cations, 20
Cerebral edema, 16–17, 58
Chlorides, normal blood concentrations, 68
Clinical teaching, 99–110
Colloid osmotic pressure, 19
Concentration gradient:
　defined, 9
　effects of diffusion on, 12
Crystalloid osmotic pressure, 15

Daily weight, 63–64
Diffusion:
　defined, 10
　effects of concentration gradients on, 10, 12
　facilitated, 12
　lipid soluble, 11
　through pores, 10
Digitalis toxicity, 48–49
Diuretics, 49
Drugs, effects of fluid and electrolytes on, 66–67

Edema:
　causes of, 17–19
　cerebral, 17, 58
　pulmonary, 18
　tissue, 19, 58
Electrolytes (nonprotein solutes):
　anions, 20
　cations, 20

Electrolytes (nonprotein solutes):
　characteristics of, 20–22
　defined, 20
　functions, 21–23
　loss of, 38–40
　measurement of, 21
　milliequivalents, 31
　observations related to, 48–50
　relationship to crystalloid osmotic pressure, 15
　renal regulation, 25
　role of acid-base balance in, 17–18
　sensory changes related to, 58–59
Extracellular fluid:
　characteristics of, 9
　composition of, 9, 21

Fluid replacement therapy, 84–89

Hematocrit, 68
Homeostasis, 42–44
Hydrogen ions, 30, 37
　normal concentrations:
　　urine, 68
　　venous, 68
　relationship to pH, 30
Hydrostatic pressure, 18–20
Hypercalcemia (see Calcium imbalance)

Hyperkalemia (see Potassium imbalance, increases in)
Hypocalcemia (see Calcium imbalance)
Hypokalemia (see Potassium imbalance, decreases in)
Hyponatremia (see Sodium imbalance, depletion of)

Immobilization, 67, 78–81
  prevention of cardiovascular effects, 79
  prevention of metabolic effects, 80
  prevention of respiratory effects, 79–80
Infants, fluid balance, 8
Intake and output:
  common errors in, 83
  role of nurse in maintenance of, 71–74
Intracellular fluid:
  characteristics of, 9
  composition of, 21
  defined, 9

Kidneys (nephron):
  effects of ADH on, 26–28
  effects of aldosterone on, 28–29
  effects of blood volume on, 30
  function, 25–30
  glomerular capillaries, 25
  glomerular filtrate, 25

Kidneys (nephron):
  sodium excretion, 30
  structure, 24–25

Metabolic acidosis, 51
Metabolic alkalosis, 51
Milliequivalents, 21

Nephron (see Kidneys)
Nonprotein solutes (see Electrolytes)
Nurse, role of:
  in assessment (see Assessment of patients)
  clinical teaching, 99–110
  communication, 82–84
  observation: of daily weight, 63–64
    of gastrointestinal output, 61–62
    of physical appearance and activity, 56–58
    of sensory status, 58–59
    of urinary output, 62–63
    of vital signs, 59–61

Orthostatic hypotension, 81
Osmosis, 13–15

pH, 30
Potassium:
  foods high in, 74
  foods low in, 77

INDEX

Potassium:
  normal blood values, 68
  renal excretion, 28, 29
  replacement, 36
Potassium imbalance:
  causes of, 3, 38
  decreases in, 48–49
  increases in, 49–50

Replacement solutions (intravenous fluids):
  hypertonic, 17–18
  hypotonic, 16–17
  isotonic, 15–16

Sodium:
  normal blood values, 68
  renal excretion, 28, 29
  replacement, 36
Sodium imbalance,
  causes of, 4–5
  depletion of, 48

Sodium imbalance:
  increases, signs of, 58
Sweat, 72
  composition of, 41
  effects of supine position on, 80

Urinalysis, normal values, 68
Urine output, 62–63

Venous gases, normal values, 68
Vital signs, 59–61

Water imbalance, causes of, 4–5
Weighing, criteria for, 64
Weight:
  attributable to water, 7
  changes in, significance of, 63–64
  relationship to hemodialysis, 77–78